—— REVISED FOURTH EDITION ——

The **Type 2**
Diabetes
Diet Book

Other books by Robert E. Kowalski

The 8-Week Cholesterol Cure

Cholesterol & Children

The 8-Week Cholesterol Cure Cookbook

8 Steps to a Healthy Heart

The Revolutionary Cholesterol Breakthrough

— REVISED FOURTH EDITION —

The Type 2 Diabetes Diet Book

CALVIN EZRIN, M.D.
ROBERT E. KOWALSKI

New York   Chicago   San Francisco   Athens   London   Madrid
Mexico City   Milan   New Delhi   Singapore   Sydney   Toronto

4 5 6 7 8 9 10 11 12 13 14 15   DOC/DOC   1 0 9 8 7 6 5 4

ISBN   978-0-07-174526-0
MHID   0-07-174526-2

e-ISBN   978-0-07-176129-1
e-MHID   0-07-176129-2

Library of Congress Cataloging-in-Publication Data

Ezrin, Calvin.

The type 2 diabetes book / Calvin Ezrin, Robert E. Kowalski.
Rev. 4th Ed.
xxiii, 247 p. : ill. ; 23 cm.
Includes bibliographical references (p. 233–235) and index.
ISBN 0-07-174526-2

1. Non-insulin-independent diabetes—Nutritional aspects—Popular works.
2. Non-insulin-independent diabetes—Diet therapy—Recipes.
3. High-protein diet. 4. Low-carbohydrate diet. 5. Insulin—Metabolism—Regulation. 6. Diabetes Mellitus, Type II—diet therapy—Popular Works.
7. Diabetic Diet—Popular Works.

RC662.18 .E97 2011
616.4620654
                                        2011377332

This book is dedicated to the memory of Robert (Bob) Kowalski, a giant in the field of medical journalism. I was privileged to know him for almost thirty years, as a collaborator on several books and as his student in the art of effective scientific writing. *The Type 2 Diabetes Diet Book* is a tribute to his capacity to express complex concepts in a warm and supportive way. He helped numerous patients, especially with cholesterol control. I will always remember him as an honorary physician. I miss him greatly.

To Gerry Ezrin, my partner in life, an outstanding wife and mother of eight, who continues to be an inspiration in all my endeavors.

The weight loss diet proposed in this book reflects an approach to weight loss that has been developed while medically supervising patients. The book has been written as a guide to be used by the patient under the supervision of his or her personal physician.

The weight loss regimen described here has been designed for use specifically for those individuals with large amounts of weight to lose—those who have been classified as medically obese. Obesity is defined as weighing at least 20 percent more than the ideal weight. Increased morbidity and mortality are associated with overweight of this magnitude.

The protein-sparing, modified-fast diet has been well documented as being safe and effective, especially for those who are significantly overweight. This book describes that type of diet; guides the reader through aspects of the dietary regimen, including food suggestions and recipes; and provides information so readers can understand the principles of this approach. By providing this information, *The Type 2 Diabetes Diet Book* can be a useful bridge between doctor and patient.

CONTENTS

PREFACE

An initial weight gain of 10 to 20 pounds is enough to set in motion progressive increases in insulin resistance that make permanent weight control very difficult. The inciting weight may be gained in various ways, for example, through stopping smoking, depression, steroid medication, or immobilization following a trauma. The accumulated excess fat produces increased amounts of adepokines, selective antagonist to the blood sugar–lowering effect of insulin, but that spares insulin's fat-building influence. To combat the rise in blood sugar, more insulin is secreted, which stimulates hunger, particularly for carbohydrates. The extra calories consumed are stored as more fat, which produces more adepokines and, thereby, more and more fat. To break this cycle, insulin must be reduced by a low calorie, low carbohydrate diet plus increased aerobic exercise.

Another important source of carbohydrate craving is a deficiency of the brain chemical serotonin. Chronic stress depletes serotonin, resulting in weight gain and sleep disturbance. Deep, restorative sleep can be achieved by serotonin supplementation with an appropriate bedtime medication such as trazodone, which creates more serotonin and in time replenishes this deficit.

The secrets of successful permanent weight loss are

1. controlling insulin through diet and exercise and
2. enhancing serotonin from good sleep.

This book shows you how to do both!

ACKNOWLEDGMENTS

To Dawn Messenger, who for many years served my practice ably as a weight counselor, I owe much gratitude. She would agree that the development of this book would have been impossible without the lessons that our patients taught us and the inspiration they engendered to share the knowledge we gained.

Grateful acknowledgment goes to Charlene Mais-Hanson for her help in revising the exercise chapter and to Kristen L. Caron, who has been an effective nutrition consultant in my practice and provided several new recipes for this edition.

Lana Temme, RD, is a highly skilled, caring, and meticulous registered dietitian whose expertise has helped the program accomplish excellent blood sugar control in our diabetic patients, as well as remarkable weight loss results in our overweight patients. She has been with us for five years and has seen and helped more than 3,000 individuals. She is also a private consultant in her own practice called Your Dietitian.

—CALVIN EZRIN, M.D.

INTRODUCTION

For decades, I have been involved in the treatment of diabetes, and I am impressed by the rapid developments in this area of health during the past few years. Never before has the medical community focused on this type of health issue with the scrutiny it recently has received.

A significant development in the field is the revised approach to diagnosing Type 2 diabetes, which is now indicated by blood sugars with a level of 126 mg/dl as compared to the previous indication level of 140 mg/dl. The cutoff point was lowered because newer research showed that even those diabetic individuals with no symptoms still develop complications, including damage to the small blood vessels throughout the body that may lead to degeneration of the kidney (nephropathy); increased risk of heart disease and stroke; and decreased blood flow to the extremities, which can necessitate amputation in worst-case scenarios. As a matter of public health, this revision in diagnostic criteria has resulted in an increase in the estimate of people with Type 2 diabetes.

In September 2008, a report by the Centers for Disease Control and Prevention indicated that there were at least 23.6 million diabetic patients in the United States, including Type 1 and Type 2 diabetics. Less than 10 percent of those afflicted were Type 1, with the remainder being Type 2 diabetics. Diabetes has approached epidemic proportions throughout the Western world, while also becoming increasingly common in developing countries. Furthermore, a recent survey showed that approximately two-thirds of American adults are now considered medically obese (at least 20 percent more than their ideal or healthy weight), a condition highly linked to Type 2 diabetes.

Obesity and Type 2 diabetes are the most common expressions of what has been called the insulin resistance syndrome. Because insulin is regulated by blood sugar levels, a rise in blood sugar calls for more insulin to bring the blood sugar to normal. This situation is called compensatory hyperinsulinism and is characteristic of a number of disorders, including Type 2 diabetes.

Though the principles and the practical suggestions in the previous edition of this book remain important and valid, this new edition contains numerous additions and changes that bring the program up-to-date. People with diabetes require medical supervision. This book will help them communicate with their physicians regarding the importance of positively controlling their blood sugar (glucose); utilizing the minimum amount of insulin, either natural or by injection; and relying on fewer or no oral prescription drugs. Only a physician can regulate the medical treatment in diabetes and thereby decide which medications may or may not be necessary.

The program presented here is a practical blend of low carbohydrate dieting plus nonintimidating exercises, both of which reduce the excess insulin that drives the accompanying obesity toward diabetes. Weight loss remains the most important and vital means of decreasing insulin resistance. By increasing sensitivity to insulin, the levels of glucose in the blood and the potential for diabetic complications are reduced. Weight loss in Type 2 diabetes has traditionally been difficult to achieve and frustrating to both patients and physicians, but success can be vastly improved with an insulin-controlled diet and an exercise program, supplemented by the benefit of good sleep from trazodone.

ANGEL AND DEMON: THE TWO FACES OF INSULIN

Insulin was discovered in my home city, Toronto, Canada, in 1921. The two men most credited with this discovery, Dr. Fred Banting and later Dr. Charles Best, would become my teachers and my inspiration when I was a medical student at the University of Toronto in the mid-1940s. In the preinsulin era, the diagnosis of diabetes in young people was a death sentence. This category of diabetes is now called Type 1, in contrast with the more common Type 2 diabetes that affects older and heavier patients. Young diabetics then could be sustained by starvation diets for three to five years but ultimately succumbed to the disease not long after. I learned about the miracle of insulin in the lecture hall with accompanying slide projections of the patients' emaciated conditions. These children, who were at death's door, were revived rapidly by insulin, which restored their blood sugars to normal, followed by healthy weight gains. With the aid of insulin, they could live a long time in relatively good health, often sixty years or more. For these young patients, insulin was regarded as an angel of mercy.

It took forty years after the discovery of insulin before it could be measured in blood. In Type 1 diabetics there was very little detectable insulin at the time of diagnosis. It had been depleted by the immune system, which destroyed the pancreatic beta cells, the source of insulin, an autoimmune disease. There were two conditions in which the blood insulin level was unexpectedly elevated, namely, obesity and Type 2 diabetes, at the time of diagnosis. In Type 2 diabetics insulin production often declines sufficiently to require insulin injections for proper control. These observations verify the important role of insulin in the pathogenesis of Type 2 diabetes.

This role of insulin in the pathogenesis of Type 2 diabetes may begin with an initial weight gain of 10 pounds (women) or 15 pounds (men) and is sufficient to initiate a process that can become independent of the events that first caused the weight increase. Examples of such events include depression, inactivity, pregnancy, smoking cessation, and use of such medications as steroids or psychotropic drugs. However, it does not matter exactly how this initial weight is gained; what is most important is that the fat is deposited predominantly in the abdomen. Once this takes place, the fat is considered toxic visceral fat, which produces negative chemicals that are released into the body's circulation. The major ill effect of visceral fat is its interference with the glucose-lowering effect of insulin. The usual amounts of insulin required to control blood glucose are no longer adequate when faced with this visceral fat, leading to an increased secretion of insulin in attempts to restore normal glycemia.

Insulin, however, can also act as a fat-building hormone, an action that is not inhibited by the toxic fat products. Not only does insulin add fat to the fat cells, but it also prevents its release. Thus, insulin can be regarded as a jailer of stored fat. Increased fat is largely deposited in the abdomen along with the original toxic reservoir, thereby sharing its malevolent properties. Thus, a metabolic trap is created that ultimately can lead to Type 2 diabetes when the demand for insulin exceeds its reserve capacity. In this setting, insulin actually can cause diabetes.

The role of insulin as a demon is revealed by this contribution to the development of Type 2 diabetes and the obesity that usually precedes it. This linkage is expressed by the term "diabesity." Low carbohydrate diets and aerobic exercise, both of which reduce insulin secretion, can help offset insulin's bad influences. However, experience has shown that these lifestyle changes, while they often succeed initially, rarely maintain their benefit, presumably because of depletion of serotonin brought on by the stress involved in pursuing these lifestyle changes.

This book does not deal much with Type 1 diabetes and the life-saving role of insulin in that disorder; instead it addresses the demonic role of insulin that characterizes Type 2 diabetes and the other insulin-resistant syndromes. The aim of diabetic patients should be to best control blood sugar with the least amount of insulin. For the other insulin-resistant states, weight loss and insulin sensitizers, such as metformin, should be the preferred response.

Once weight control is managed through the benefits of exercise, diet, and restorative sleep with the aid of trazodone, patients can expect to greatly lessen the accompanying degenerative diseases including heart disease, stroke, and diabetic complications. While the data substantiating such hopes are not yet available, there are strong indications that remaining at a healthy weight also pays off by reducing the risk of many types of cancers, including uterine, breast, and colon.

Moreover, there is the far more immediate and personal satisfaction one enjoys merely by looking in the mirror and fitting into clothes previously relegated to the back of the closet. Then, too, those successfully following this program feel more vibrant and energetic, sleep more soundly and restfully, and are more satisfied with themselves and their lives.

And so, without any further ado, I eagerly welcome you to this revised edition of *The Type 2 Diabetes Diet Book* and the Insulin Control Diet.

GOOD SLEEP WILL MAKE ONE THIN

There is no denying the continuing increases in obesity and Type 2 diabetes. In the United States, this situation has become an epidemic threatening to overwhelm our health care budget. Approximately 66 percent (two-thirds) of the U.S. adult population is currently, or has been, overweight. Every increase in weight of 11 pounds (5 kilograms) increases the risk of developing diabetes by 4.5 percent. Approximately 83 percent of people with Type 2 diabetes in the United States are either overweight or obese. In 2007 the cost of diabetes in the United States was calculated to be $174 billion, of which one-half was for inpatient treatment of diabetes and its complications.

Experience has taught us that weight loss is the best prescription for preventing or reversing Type 2 diabetes, but it is difficult to sustain. Numerous studies have been unable to find a measurable abnormality that would account for the almost universal failure of weight loss diets to maintain their initial success. Is there an organ in the body that does not communicate with the bloodstream, making it impossible to measure an underlying abnormality in blood tests that might account for this failure?

The answer is yes—the brain. It sits in the skull covered by the blood-brain barrier, which prevents the escape into the circulation of its controlling chemicals (forty neurotransmitters). Since it is generally agreed that the brain is the dominant organ in the body, ultimately regulating all other systems, these neurotransmitters actually control the brain. One of them, serotonin, regulates the other thirty-nine by promoting deep, restorative sleep. Thus, serotonin can be considered the most important neurotransmitter. Through animal studies, it appears that normal mental and physical activities throughout the day result in a reduction of neurotransmitters, which is corrected by good restorative sleep, especially in regard to the amount of serotonin present. As long as there is enough serotonin, all will be well. What if there is insufficient serotonin, and why does this occur? Stress from a variety of causes brings worrisome thoughts that impair the sleep process and decrease serotonin replenishment. Two symptoms then emerge: carbohydrate cravings and daytime fatigue.

It is imperative to stress that sleep deprivation is a key weight control component that has not received the attention it deserves. Americans sleep the least of modern countries' citizens, and they are the most overweight and obese. Dr. Eve VanCaughter, a sleep researcher at the University of Chicago, has written that sleep should be included in any intervention for weight loss. About one-third of the U.S. population experiences disrupted sleep, which includes problems falling asleep, the inability to stay asleep, and failure to feel restored by sleep. In many subjects, sleep is so dysfunctional that it impairs daytime performance. Daytime fatigue, particularly in the late afternoon, is a reliable indicator of poor quality sleep. When stress impairs the depth and restorative quality of sleep, serotonin is depleted and carbohydrate cravings emerge. Many such patients describe themselves as "carboholics" because of their uncontrollable addictions to simple carbohydrates.

Insulin has an important role in the pathogenesis and treatment of obesity and Type 2 diabetes. Its major actions are to decrease glucose by increasing its utilization and storage and to increase the buildup of fat. Another aspect of insulin, however, that is usually overlooked is it decreases amino acids with the exception of L-tryptophan, the precursor of serotonin. Since the blood-brain barrier has a limited number of openings that allow the entry of amino acids into the brain, there is a strong competition among the twenty-two amino acids to get into the central nervous system. No amino acid has any advantage over another, except in the case where insulin acts to spare L-tryptophan and reduce all of the other competing amino acids at the same time. Comfort foods are rapidly digested, raising blood sugar and insulin, which allows the production of a small amount of serotonin. The comfort and contentment produced by serotonin lasts only a short time, but the increased carbohydrate-related calories remain and increase fat stores. The comfort induced by simple carbohydrates fuels the addiction and ultimately may lead to obesity and Type 2 diabetes.

Effort is often directed at decreasing insulin's malevolent influence through low carbohydrate diets and aerobic exercise, which reduce insulin secretion. While these lifestyle changes often succeed initially, they rarely achieve lasting benefits, likely because of the depletion of serotonin brought on by the stress involved in pursuing these demanding changes.

Trazodone is a well-tolerated sedative-hypnotic and a serotonin agonist that provides a jump-start for the sleep process, supporting a deep restorative level that increases serotonin and the other thirty-nine neurotransmitters. Trazodone should be considered for patients who may admit to or exhibit carbohydrate cravings and daytime fatigue. Ideally, use of trazodone should be initiated at the start of the weight loss program so that the improved sleep and control of cravings generated will make it easier to adhere to a restricted calorie or low carbohydrate diet, while providing additional energy throughout the day.

Since the dose of trazodone required to achieve these benefits can vary greatly by patient, the starting dose should be low and increased slowly. Begin with 25 milligrams of trazodone one-half hour before bedtime for one week and then raise it by 25–50 milligrams weekly until daytime energy is restored and cravings are abolished. In a few patients, as much as 500 milligrams may be needed. The low carbohydrate diet program outlined in this book, along with its exercise recommendations, will provide the nutritional and behavioral advice required for sustained weight loss. When a reasonable goal weight has been reached, the patient is ready for the next phase: stabilization. This step involves a gradual increase in calories and carbohydrates until caloric equilibrium is achieved. Then, in a longer-lasting maintenance phase, the trazodone dose should be held fairly constant for three to six months to restore the brain's serotonin sufficiently, followed by gradual withdrawal at monthly intervals. If during this time either the symptoms of daytime fatigue or carbohydrate cravings recur, the withdrawal should be temporarily halted and the former effective dose reinitiated for one or two months to increase cerebral serotonin. Then, the dose reduction can be resumed.

Trazodone is generally well tolerated with only minor side effects, such as dry mouth and constipation, which easily can be overcome. Check for postural hypotension that may emerge, particularly if salt is restricted. Priapism is very rare and should not be feared. When the successful withdrawal of trazodone is complete, providing adequate serotonin from good sleep is now the responsibility of the brain, which takes over from the medication.

Trazodone is a uniquely safe and effective medication that makes itself less and less necessary over time and, ultimately, unnecessary after a satisfactory weight loss. Followed somewhat later by a gradual withdrawal of trazodone under supervision, this ideal state can be maintained by simple measures that need not involve the medication. Patients are advised to weigh themselves weekly. If as little as 5 pounds are gained, the low carbohydrate, ketogenic diet should be resumed until this surplus weight is lost, usually within three weeks, and then followed by a return to the maintenance diet. Waiting for a further increase in weight before taking such action makes weight gain harder to control without trazodone. However, if needed in the future, this medication can help once again.

TRAZODONE AS A SLEEP AID AND WEIGHT LOSS DRUG

Trazodone has been criticized as lacking high-quality research data on its ability to help people sleep. What is left unsaid is that because trazodone is no longer patented, no pharmaceutical company stands to profit from doing such research (Carlat D. *New York Times* Op-Ed May 9, 2006). Trazodone is approved by the Food and Drug Administration (FDA) as a high dose antidepressant but is more commonly used "off label" as a lower dose sleep aid. Prescribing trazodone may be the most frequent "off label" use of a drug in all of psychopharmacology. "Off label" means that the FDA has not approved the medication for this therapeutic use, but the term does not imply that prescribing trazodone for this purpose is a bad thing. The FDA regulates the sale of medicine, not the practice of medicine, and does not forbid the use of trazodone as a sleep aid. The practice of medicine is set instead by community standards of care, experts, and guidelines. In clinical practice, trazodone has become accepted as the most popular sleep aid in the United States. With continued favorable experience and results, trazodone should become equally popular in its use as a weight loss drug.

Because of the extreme importance of replenishing serotonin with bedtime trazodone at the beginning of weight loss treatment, the medication should be prescribed along with diet and exercise advice. The major unmet challenge in the treatment of obesity and related Type 2 diabetes (diabesity) is to provide sustained weight loss. My intention is to share with physicians my experience with serotonin replenishment, the lack of which is responsible for the onset of obesity and later failure to maintain weight loss by diet and exercise alone.

The benefits of this program are many. The risks are negligible, and the efforts required are moderate. The necessary partnership between the diabetic patient and supervising physician will be strengthened by the communication required to make this program work optimally.

Chapter 1

THE CRITICAL ROLE OF DIET IN DIABETES

The first recorded diagnosis of diabetes was made by physicians in ancient Egypt. Finding that the urine of patients with the disease tasted sweet, they named the problem *mellitus* meaning "honey."

Diabetes remains defined as a disease characterized by elevated levels of blood sugar, glucose, caused by a relative deficiency of the hormone insulin. There are two major types of the disease.

The less common, insulin-dependent diabetes mellitus, or *Type 1 diabetes*, occurs mainly in the young. For that reason it was previously called juvenile diabetes. Accounting for about 10 percent of all cases, Type 1 results from a near total destruction of the beta cells of the pancreas that make insulin. Type 1 is often initiated by a virus attack and a subsequent malfunctioning of the body's own immune system that destroys the cells of the pancreas that produce insulin. Type 1 diabetes patients are rarely overweight at the onset of their illnesses, but they can gain weight easily owing to the insulin treatment required for survival.

The more common, second form of this endocrine disturbance is noninsulin-dependent diabetes mellitus, now termed *Type 2 diabetes*. It is not associated with insulin deficiency but rather with a substantial resistance to the hormone's blood sugar–lowering effect. Most typically, Type 2 develops in adulthood and was previously known as *maturity-onset diabetes*. Often Type 2 diabetes patients have normal or even increased levels of insulin in their blood but not in sufficient amounts to keep the blood sugar within normal limits. About 90 percent of these patients are obese in medical terms.

Diet has been linked with diabetes from the beginning, and it remains a critical component of treatment today. In fact, an understanding of how dietary management influences the disease is the first step in controlling it.

INSULIN RESISTANCE AND HYPERINSULINISM

While the overweight condition of diabetes patients is at least partially the result of poor eating habits, the phenomena of insulin resistance and hyperinsulinism promote weight gain and make weight loss particularly difficult. Thus, most efforts at weight control for Type 2 diabetics are frustrating and ultimately end in failure. Only when the factors of insulin resistance and hyperinsulinism are taken into consideration can one expect to succeed.

What causes insulin resistance? In Type 2 diabetes it is a strongly inherited selective defect in blood sugar regulation. This affects muscle predominantly but also involves the liver and fat tissue.

Insulin is necessary to metabolize glucose for the body to use it as fuel in the cells. But in diabetic patients, glucose resists this action of insulin. Viewed another way, the insulin is less capable of metabolizing glucose in the diabetic patient than those without diabetes. In response, the body produces additional insulin in an effort to metabolize the rising levels of sugar in the blood. Ultimately, an excessive level of insulin results, a condition termed *hyperinsulinism.*

For a time, the additional insulin may be sufficient to maintain relatively normal blood sugar levels. But this is a catch-22 situation. Increased insulin levels favor a gain in fat weight, which, in turn, is another important cause of insulin resistance. Fat tissue produces severe chemicals (adipokines) that inhibit the muscles' ability to utilize glucose as fuel or for storage as glycogen.

There comes a time when sufficient weight is gained so that the combined forms of insulin resistance exceed the ability of the pancreas to respond with adequate insulin secretion. At that point, the person is diagnosed with diabetes. Research indicates that a Type 2 diabetes patient has a subtle defect in the pancreas's ultimate ability to make as much insulin as can a nondiabetic individual, whose pancreas has considerable potential reserve capacity. Often, however, excess insulin also produces diabetics who may then require insulin control, starting with diet and exercise as treatment.

Even in the nondiabetic, insulin is involved with production of the "bad" cholesterol carrier known as low-density lipoproteins, or LDL.

At the same time, insulin lowers levels of the "good" cholesterol carrier, high-density lipoproteins (HDL), and strongly stimulates growth of certain cells that play pivotal roles in arterial disease. Imagine, then, what can happen when excessive amounts of insulin circulate through the blood. All those negative functions are increased tremendously. This connection explains some of the reasons why diabetes patients are at significantly greater risk of heart disease and other cardiovascular complications so common in diabetics.

Interestingly, while we typically think of insulin in positive terms, there is a dark side to this hormone.

The landmark Diabetes Control and Complications Trial showed conclusively that good blood sugar control led to significantly better outcomes. That is, Type 1 patients who had "tight control" over their glucose levels suffered fewer complications involving the eyes, nerves, kidneys, and blood vessels. Since Type 2 diabetics develop similar complications, it was reasonable to conclude that good control of blood sugar would be equally desirable for them as well. In the case of small blood vessel–related complications this is true. But regarding large vessel events such as heart disease, stroke, and gangrene, there is some concern that the extra insulin required for good control may be harmful.

Both high blood sugars and high blood insulin levels are likely contributors to Type 2 diabetes large vessel complications. Ideally, levels of sugar and insulin should be normalized. This, happily enough, can be done by following the weight control program detailed in this book.

Excessive secretion of insulin is invariably higher in obese individuals than their lean counterparts. Both obese and lean individuals will release additional insulin in response to meals. But the more obese the individual, the more elevated the plasma insulin.

Those with the lowest fasting insulin have the greatest blood sugar response to insulin; those with the highest fasting insulin have insulin resistance. Again, the higher the level of obesity, the greater the insulin resistance in women and men of all ages, in a linear fashion. This levels off as one becomes very obese.

Insulin metabolizes sugar, making it available to the body's cells. But it also restricts metabolism of fat, leading to fat storage. Hence the obese have less release of free fatty acids and less breakdown of fats, a process known as *lipolysis*. However, certain fat cells are resistant to the hormone (lypes) that prevents the release of fatty acids, which leads to triglyceride overproduction, the largest found in Type 2 diabetics.

The link between obesity and high blood pressure has long been noted in medicine. Now we know that this is due to insulin resistance; there is a high prevalence of hypertension in insulin-resistant individuals. Indeed, it is possible to actually measure the influence of weight on blood pressure. For every pound (2.2 kilograms) of weight gained in excess of one's healthy weight, blood pressure goes up 0.2 to 0.3 mm/Hg (millimeters of mercury on the doctor's blood pressure meter).

WEIGHT CONTROL AND DIABETES

Weight control from a low carbohydrate diet and a reasonable program of physical exercise are the two most critical components of effective diabetes management. Since most Type 2 diabetics are overweight, the diet prescribed should be low in calories so that stored fat must be withdrawn to provide the calories no longer provided by the food.

> Think of fat as a potential food source—your body's pantry.

Let's run that by one more time, since it is such an important concept. The excess weight you have takes the form of stored fat. Your body needs a certain amount of fuel on a daily basis—energy measured in calories. Reduce the number of calories and the body can turn to that "pantry" to make up the deficit. Unfortunately, that ideal scenario doesn't always occur in the typical weight loss diet. But, fortunately, that's exactly what happens in the program you're now reading about.

What are some of the particulars about an ideal diet for the diabetic patient? There is no argument among the world's authorities that sufficient protein must be included to provide the essential amino acids that the body cannot synthesize. A low-protein diet would be prescribed only if the patient has kidney disease.

Now what about carbohydrates and fat, the remaining two potential sources of energy? High carbohydrate diets produce higher plasma glucose and insulin levels. Obviously from what we've already discussed, that's defeating the purpose. Moreover, such diets generate significantly higher triglycerides and lower HDL levels, especially when compared to this book's program. A diet low in carbohydrates prevents those adverse responses. On this program, blood sugar and insulin levels fall dramatically, as does the level of triglycerides. A beneficial state of ketosis (described later in this chapter) appears within two to three days, indicating that insulin levels have been sufficiently reduced to allow fat to be rapidly mobilized from the body's stores to provide a major source of energy.

As a direct result of returning to a healthy weight and controlling excessive amounts of insulin, one can expect to achieve a normal glucose level. Type 2 diabetes, in fact, is diagnosed in terms of glucose levels in excess of 126 mg/dl. But today there is a measurement considered the gold standard for monitoring how your body utilizes glucose. This standard is glycosylated hemoglobin (Hba1c), pronounced H-B-A-one-C, or hemoglobin A-one-C.

Glycosylated hemoglobin measures the average blood sugar of the preceding two to three months. It is much more informative than isolated blood sugars and is now the measure by which your doctor will judge the excellence of control of diabetes.

In addition to carrying oxygen in the blood, hemoglobin binds glucose to a degree that is determined by the height of the blood sugar level and the duration of any elevation. There is a normal range of binding that is exceeded in diabetics unless they are under excellent control. I call this test "sugar-coated hemoglobin."

It is particularly useful in tracking control of diabetes because the red blood cells that carry hemoglobin in the blood are recycled every three months. The new red cells carry fresh hemoglobin that will reflect only the blood sugars of the following three months.

By following the program outlined here, you'll keep dietary fat to a minimum in order to maximize the withdrawal of internal fat. You might be asked how many calories you're consuming on your diet. The correct answer would be 2,000 calories. Imagine the response you'd get to that reply. "What! How can you lose weight on 2,000 calories?" The answer is that only 1,000 of those calories come from the food you eat, while 1,000 calories are supplied by your stored fat—from your body's pantry.

Diabetes and Heart Disease

Heart disease remains the number one cause of death in the United States. It is an equal opportunity killer, taking the lives of literally half of all men and women. Although women enjoy some special protection earlier in life, they quickly catch up with and exceed male rates of heart attacks and death after menopause.

> Exercise is the best "drug" for insulin resistance.

Cholesterol levels are particularly important for diabetics. Type 2 diabetics are at special risk when levels are low for the protective HDL cholesterol and high for triglycerides and LDL cholesterol. The risk of death, as published in the journal *Circulation,* was four times as great and the chances of having any cardiac event was two times as high for such individuals.

While diabetes has long been recognized as a particularly dangerous risk factor for heart disease, the focus has now narrowed to the insulin resistance that accompanies diabetes. Type 2 patients have elevated levels of glucose in the blood since their insulin is unable to facilitate the use of that blood sugar by the cells. As a result, their bodies produce additional insulin to compensate, leading to the condition known as *hyperinsulinemia.* But such individuals are insulin resistant, and even excessive levels may not decrease sugar loads. Now doctors are recognizing that those excessive insulin levels are at least partially responsible for the diabetic patient's increased risk of heart disease.

Insulin resistance is accompanied by a constellation of risks, including elevated triglycerides, lowered HDL counts, and high blood pressure. Previously, some doctors believed that it was those accompanying factors that were responsible for the added risk. Now the higher-than-normal levels of insulin in the blood are seen as dangerous.

Testing for insulin resistance is not commonly performed, as it is both expensive and time-consuming. To do so, doctors administer glucose and insulin intravenously over at least three hours to determine how much insulin is required to maintain a constant normal level of blood sugar. This is called the glucose clamp technique. Results are fed into a computer that calculates the body's response to the insulin.

Further aggravating the problem, some medications used to treat high blood pressure and to correct cholesterol and other lipid elevations actually result in raising insulin levels. And, in some cases, when diabetic patients are unable to control glucose levels through diet, exercise, and oral medications, doctors prescribe insulin injections to lower the sugar counts. That extra insulin may lead to increased heart disease risk.

Approximately twenty-four million Americans have diabetes. It is often said that half of all diabetics remain undiagnosed. Diabetes is the fourth leading cause of death in the United States. Because of damage done by diabetes to nerve endings, patients may not sense the symptoms of heart disease, such as chest pain, and the disease goes untreated and worsens. Moreover, diabetic patients suffer from impaired function of the left ventricle of the heart, the pumping chamber. Such individuals benefit from drugs such as aspirin, beta blockers, and angiotensin-converting enzyme (ACE) inhibitors and ACE receptor blockers, more than those without diabetes.

What are the practical implications of all this? Obviously, it behooves people with diabetes to work diligently toward tight control of glucose levels and reductions of insulin in their blood. For those with Type 2 diabetes, weight control and regular exercise along with good sleep from trazodone can be virtually miraculous, leading to the practical elimination of disease manifestations in most cases.

Women, Weight, and Waists

Women must not only worry about excess weight but also about the size of their waists. And it's not just a matter of vanity. Large waists increase a woman's risk of Type 2 diabetes. The more overweight a woman becomes, the higher her risk, and simply measuring the waist is an accurate predictor of danger.

When compared with women whose waists average 28 inches, risk increases by two and a half times for those with a 30- or 31-inch waist. It jumps to four times the risk for those with a 32- or 33-inch waist, and six times the average risk for women whose waists measure 38 inches or larger.

The greater the risk for diabetes, the greater the risk for heart disease. So, by inference, waist size also can predict the risk of heart disease. This is in keeping with previous research showing that those with "apple" shapes (excess weight around the waist) are at greater risk than individuals with "pear" shapes (weight distributed more in the hips and thighs).

Not Just Heart Disease, but Also Stroke

Obese women, or those who have gained more than 44 pounds since age eighteen, are at two and a half times the risk of stroke than those who have not gained weight since they were younger. Those findings come from Brigham and Women's Hospital in Boston.

The combination of health, diet, and weight control follows a kind of domino concept. First comes the weight gain, caused most typically by overeating and sedentary behavior, followed by a waterfall of degenerative diseases, including diabetes, heart disease, and stroke. The good news is that by taking care of the weight, as this book will show you how to do, you'll automatically control those other fronts as well.

KETOSIS AS PART OF WEIGHT LOSS

For many years now, health professionals have known how to feed seriously ill patients intravenously. A specially developed formula that includes emulsified fat is fed directly into the vein, and this emulsified fat can be used immediately as energy for the body.

Needless to say, if any other kind of fat—including the fat stored in your own body—were injected directly into the vein, the results would be disastrous. But imagine how efficient it would be if your body's fat were to be rendered so it could be used directly as energy. That's exactly what happens when following this program, as your body enters a state of mild, beneficial ketosis.

Obviously, the first benefit would be the loss of the weight stored as fat. But there are additional advantages to ketosis. You'll experience appetite control without the overstimulation of the nervous system that so often occurs when taking diet pills. Those pills also produce despondency and depression never seen with ketosis. Next, ketosis induces a gentle diuresis characterized by a selective excretion of sodium and water while at the same time sparing potassium, and without the significant rebound resistance that occurs with diuretic pills. Finally, ketosis spares protein by substituting for glucose as brain fuel, thereby limiting the amount of new glucose that must be made from amino acids, the building blocks of protein.

There are two types of ketosis, one good and the other bad. It is crucial that both you and your doctor know the difference. The good ketosis just described results from the reduction of insulin, sufficient to permit rapid liberation of fatty acids from stored fat and their subsequent conversion in the liver. This results in moderate amounts of ketones that are never sufficient enough to disturb the chemical acid-base balance of the body. The ketosis advocated in this program never produces acidosis.

The bad ketosis is an acute complication of diabetes usually occurring in Type 1 patients who are not receiving sufficient insulin. Physicians may rarely see the condition in Type 2 diabetic individuals whose insulin needs have been greatly increased due to infection or other severe stress. In such cases, blood sugar is usually quite high, often more than 400 milligrams. In severe cases the patient is dehydrated, acidotic, drowsy, and even comatose.

It is generally easy to distinguish between good and bad ketosis early on in a Type 2 diabetes patient. Beneficial ketosis is accompanied by near-normal blood sugar. Adverse ketosis, on the other hand, results in a high blood sugar from an obvious associated reason. It is unusual for this to happen in Type 2 patients. In fact, Type 2 diabetes has been called *nonketotic diabetes* because most patients, even with very high blood sugars, show little or no signs of the condition. This is because fat cells remain very sensitive to insulin's inhibitory effect on the breakdown and liberation of stored fat. The production of ketones by the liver requires rapid mobilization of free fatty acids from fat sources, which even a small amount of insulin can still prevent.

STABILIZING AND MAINTAINING WEIGHT LOSS

You'll be learning the details of the actual dietary program throughout the book, and they are the same for diabetic and nondiabetic individuals. But there are special considerations in stabilization and maintenance recommendations for Type 2 diabetics.

As a diabetic, you retain resistance to insulin even after weight loss has reduced the additional insulin resistance derived from obesity itself. As such, you may not have the same tolerance for carbohydrates that nondiabetics have. Your ultimate maintenance diet, required for optimal blood sugar control, should contain somewhat fewer carbohydrates. Remaining calories may come from "good" fats such as canola oil and olive oil, those that do not adversely affect cholesterol levels as do the saturated fats.

EXERCISE FOR TYPE 2 DIABETICS

Exercise is important for every man and woman to promote good health and well-being. But it is even more important for the Type 2 diabetes patient as a crucial, indispensible factor in the treatment equation.

Exercise lowers blood sugar without involving insulin. It is, therefore, a wonderful means of reducing the amount of insulin to which the body is exposed. Exercise also increases the mass of lean muscle tissue in your body, and it is that muscle that burns energy most efficiently.

What is the best fuel for exercise? Muscle contraction is fueled by a physiologic reaction involving the chemical adenosine triphosphate (ATP) as it is broken down into the metabolite adenosine diphosphate (ADP) with a resultant release of energy. Adenosine triphosphate can be derived equally well from the breakdown of glucose and fatty acids. In fact, the preferred muscle fuel for aerobic exercise is fatty acids. So much for the common misconception that the body requires carbohydrate for energy. The only time your body needs to be fueled by carbohydrates is during a marathon race or when running a 100-yard dash. You might ask yourself how likely it will be that you'll be involved in either event in the near future!

Indeed, recent studies have shown—to virtually everyone's delight—that a brisk walk is superior to jogging or running for burning fat. The reason, as we've just seen, is that the body prefers fats for fuel during such activity, as compared to burning glucose while engaged in more strenuous exercise.

After years of preaching about the advantages of strenuous exercise, something very few people are either willing or able to do, new guidelines were published. Recent guidelines simply urge all men and women to become physically active. This might mean walking around the block, taking a regular bicycle ride, doing some gardening and yard work, or taking the stairs rather than the elevator. These activities are just as effective as a structured exercise program in the gym.

For the Type 2 diabetic patient, as for the person without diabetes, the best exercise is a regular program of walking. Of course, any form of mild exercise you prefer is just fine. The important thing is that you do it regularly. Bike riding, swimming, and aerobics classes are terrific as integral components of the program.

Chapter 2

IN SEARCH OF IDEAL WEIGHT

*I was anywhere from 25 to 50 pounds
overweight for the past twenty years. Then
I discovered this wonderful program! Now I
have no more tummy. I am forty years
old, and I got back the body I had at
twenty years of age.*
—C.A., BALTIMORE, MARYLAND

Taste in physical beauty, particularly female beauty, varies widely from culture to culture and through time. In our fickle society one has to consult popular magazines to determine what this season's "ideal" figure is. The 1960s high-fashion passion for thinness has given way to a trend toward the "healthy" look, although the definition of what looks healthy comes down, once again, to personal opinion. Is the ideal body lean, flat, and smooth? Is it muscular with bulging biceps and triceps? Or does it have softer, fuller curves? At each swing of the fashion pendulum, some of us are luckier than others in terms of having the "right" appearance.

But should a person follow any standard other than his or her own in determining ideal weight? Clearly, the social pressure to be thin, especially on women, has led many down the unhealthy path of eating disorders, such as anorexia and bulimia, and to skewed perceptions of body image. But there are important reasons, quite apart from the dictates of fashion and appearance, to avoid being overweight. Medical authorities agree that excess weight is counter to good health.

THE MEDICAL CONSEQUENCES OF OBESITY

The effects of overweight are greatest during the younger years, and the longer a person is overweight, the greater the influence of this condition on ultimate longevity. It takes about ten years to develop problems associated with obesity. In later years we don't see as much influence, probably because vulnerable obese individuals have died off, leaving the hardy survivors to make up the statistics.

A 130-pound, small-framed woman who should weigh 100 pounds is considered medically obese, as is a 195-pound, average-framed man who should weigh 150 pounds.

But problems begin even before a person is clinically obese. A man who is just 10 percent overweight (for example, 165 pounds rather than the ideal 150 pounds) is at risk of increased mortality and morbidity. For a woman, risk begins to become significant at 20 percent overweight. As the weight increases, so does the risk. Mortality climbs to twelve times normal in the twenty-five- to thirty-five-year-old man at twice his ideal body weight. Thus one sees few elderly men at that degree of obesity.

How Does Obesity Kill?

Certainly the risk of heart disease, our nation's number one killer, increases as weight increases. And being overweight increases all other risk factors by two. Thus, whatever a person's increased risk is due to elevated cholesterol, that risk is doubled if the person is also overweight.

Medical obesity is 20 percent or more above ideal body weight.

Interestingly, where those extra pounds are stored on the body can also make a difference. The typical male pattern of overweight—potbelly and spare tire—associates clearly with increased risk of heart disease. The same holds true for women who put weight on in this pattern. A more evenly distributed fat layer over the entire body does not have this statistical correlation with heart disease. But, regardless of the pattern of distribution, as one increases the percentage of overweight from 10 percent to 20 percent to 30 percent and up, the risk of disease increases.

The relative risk of hypertension for overweight American adults age twenty to seventy-five years is 5.6 times that of nonoverweight persons in the same age and sex groups. Compared to obese African-American men and women, overweight Caucasian men and women are at greater risk of being hypertensive.

At the very least, any weight loss results in a drop in blood pressure, and every millimeter of difference in blood pressure means a difference in the risk of heart disease and stroke. In addition, weight loss frequently means that patients can decrease the amount of hypertension medications they take, thus diminishing any unpleasant side effects the drugs may entail.

A return to normal weight in hypertensives frequently means a return to normal blood pressure.

By now almost everyone in the nation has heard of the importance of maintaining a low level of cholesterol in the blood. It is no longer a matter of controversy: Every 1 percent drop in cholesterol means a 2 percent decrease in the risk of heart disease.

The relationship between weight and blood cholesterol level is an interesting one. Some individuals can be lean and still have a dangerously high cholesterol level; others can be stout and yet have an acceptable level. (The only way to check the cholesterol level is a simple blood test.) But the majority of overweight people experience a rise in the amount of cholesterol in their blood. Statistically speaking, overweight Americans age twenty to seventy-five have a 1.5 times greater risk of having high cholesterol. Those age twenty to forty-five have a 2.1 times greater risk. *Overweight individuals who do have elevated cholesterol levels are likely to see those levels fall if they return to normal weight.*

The same applies to the fatty substances in the blood known as *triglycerides*, which respond well to weight loss. Triglycerides, a form of fat that is abundant in the diet and also synthesized from carbohydrates, circulate in the blood until they can be used by the body. They may also contribute to atherosclerosis.

More than 80 percent of diabetics are obese. For overweight adults age twenty to seventy-five the risk of having diabetes is nearly three times that for nonoverweight adults of comparable age and sex. For those age twenty to forty-five, the risk of having diabetes is nearly four times that for nonoverweight people. Type 2, or non-insulin-dependent, diabetes (previously known as maturity-onset diabetes) is closely related to obesity. While it's true that some men and women are genetically predisposed to develop Type 2 diabetes in their mature years, the disease usually does not manifest without the development of obesity. It's as simple as that. Conversely, if an individual has Type 2 diabetes and is overweight, *simply returning to normal weight usually means that blood sugar can be controlled with fewer or no medications*. Following the program in these pages may lead to virtual reversal of the disease.

Heart disease is four times more common in those with diabetes than in the general population. For diabetic patients, weight and cholesterol control are crucial. But beyond heart disease, stroke, and diabetes, the obese person faces other risks. For example, the man weighing twice his ideal weight has a twelve times greater risk of dying from accidents than the man at his ideal weight. Due to the strain on weight-bearing joints, the incidence of arthritis skyrockets in those who are overweight. Obesity is an important risk factor for osteoarthritis of the knee, particularly in women. Obese women seem to be at greater risk of developing cancer of the uterus, colon, and breast.

Medical data clearly point to the importance of maintaining ideal weight, but the next question to be considered is what is ideal weight. How is *overweight* defined? Even in medical circles the standards used have varied through time.

The height-weight tables issued by insurance companies are the most frequently cited standards. Insurance companies determined as early as the turn of the twentieth century that excessive weight is linked with shortened life expectancies.* Not surprisingly, they began to charge more to insure obese individuals.

---

*In 1913 the Medico-Actuarial Mortality Investigation revealed that in the years from 1885 to 1909 the lowest mortality rates among insured persons were those for people whose weight was slightly above average in the younger years of adulthood and slightly below average in the older years. Bear in mind that in those years, tuberculosis and pneumonia were leading causes of death, and those diseases are associated with underweight. But a few years later, after 1913, additional studies conducted by insurance companies showed that maximum longevity was associated with weights somewhat below average.

The Metropolitan Life Insurance Company developed the first tables listing desirable weight in the early 1940s. The tables were revised in 1959, when for the first time weight standards varied according to height. (See Table 2.1.) While a number of tables have appeared since then, most are modeled after that 1959 chart. In a 1983 revision of the chart, weights were adjusted upward, which created a flurry of comments, letters, and articles in medical journals. After the dust cleared, the general consensus was that the weights proposed in the 1959 edition were more likely to be associated with better health and greater longevity.

One rule of thumb used for determining ideal body weight for men is 106 pounds for the first 5 feet of height and 6 pounds for each inch after 5 feet, plus or minus 10 percent according to frame size. The rule for women is 100 pounds for the first 5 feet, and 5 pounds per inch thereafter, with the same adjustment for frame size.

But weight alone doesn't give a completely accurate picture. More important than whether one is overweight is whether one is overfat. Think about a football player who is 6 feet tall and weighs 220 pounds. According to the standard tables he would be overweight. But is he overfat? Closer analysis would probably reveal that he is heavily muscled and has minimal body fat. On the other hand, a young girl who is underweight according to the height-weight tables might actually be overfat. The athletically conditioned person is likely to have a lower percentage of body fat than a sedentary person of identical age, sex, and genetic predisposition. And men tend to be lower in fat than women. That's just a biological fact of life.

> Lean muscle tissue is the body's engine. Only the activity of muscle can burn appreciable calories.

The body is made up primarily of bone, muscle, and fat. We can't do anything about the weight or size of our bones, but the amount of muscle and fat and the ratio between the two can change appreciably. That ratio can and does change for practically everyone through the years. The man who participated in college sports and whose body fat was on the low side can gradually lose muscle tissue and replace it with fat cells. For a long time there may be no perceptible difference. The size of his body, the girth of his waist, and even his total weight may remain the same. But his

Table 2.1 Desirable Weights for Men and Women

Height (with shoes)	Weight, in indoor clothing (lbs)		
	Small Frame	Medium Frame	Large Frame
Men			
5'2"	112–120	118–129	126–141
5'3"	115–123	121–133	129–144
5'4"	118–126	124–136	132–148
5'5"	121–129	127–139	135–152
5'6"	124–133	130–143	138–156
5'7"	128–137	134–147	142–161
5'8"	132–141	138–152	147–166
5'9"	136–145	142–156	151–170
5'10"	140–150	146–160	155–174
5'11"	144–154	150–165	159–179
6'0"	148–158	154–170	164–184
6'1"	152–162	158–175	168–189
6'2"	156–167	162–180	173–194
6'3"	160–171	167–185	178–199
6'4"	164–175	172–190	182–204
Women			
4'10"	92– 98	96–107	104–119
4'11"	94–101	98–110	106–122
5'0"	96–104	101–113	109–125
5'1"	99–107	104–116	112–128
5'2"	102–110	107–119	115–131
5'3"	105–113	110–122	118–134
5'4"	108–116	113–126	121–138
5'5"	111–119	116–130	125–142
5'6"	114–123	120–135	129–146
5'7"	118–127	124–139	133–150
5'8"	122–131	128–143	137–154
5'9"	126–135	132–147	141–158
5'10"	130–140	136–151	145–163
5'11"	134–144	140–155	149–168
6'0"	138–148	144–159	153–173

Source: Prepared by the Metropolitan Life Insurance Company. Derived primarily from data of the *Build and Blood Pressure Study,* 1959, Society of Actuaries.

muscle mass tends to atrophy. He continues to consume the same number of calories as always, noting that his weight hasn't changed a bit. He might even brag about his ability to pack away the food while still fitting into the jeans he wore at school. But one day the equation swings in favor of the fat over the lean. And, faster than he could dream possible, he begins to put weight on. He ascribes this to the inexorable passage of years. But that's not at all the reality.

To grasp the significance of body composition, we have to understand the dynamics of fat and muscle. Fat tissue cannot contribute to the burning of calories. The more lean muscle tissue one has, the more calories can be burned. As one loses that muscle tissue, the capacity to burn calories diminishes. Since fewer calories are being burned while the caloric intake remains the same, there are excess calories, and those excess calories get turned into fat. And since fat can burn no significant calories, more fat just keeps piling up, until the "spare tire" and "love handles" appear.

In this regard people are not much different from beef cattle. To get the desired well-marbled prime beef, farmers feed their livestock plenty of grain while restricting their movement. Take a look at a prime steak in the supermarket, with its white streaks of fat running through the red muscle. That's what the flesh of an overfat human looks like.

Two principal ways to determine body fat are being used today. The more accurate method is underwater weighing. The person to be weighed gets on a specially designed scale and is lowered into a pool of water. The buoyant fat does not register on the scale; only the bone and muscle get weighed. A simple calculation determines the percentage of body fat weight in relation to total body weight.

Not nearly as accurate, but a lot more convenient and adequate for many purposes, are skinfold measurements, which can be made by a trained professional. Calipers are used to measure the folds of fat at different sites on the body, principally the skinfold hanging from the underside of the arm at the triceps muscle.

Table 2.2 Suggested Standards of Fat Percentage for Adult Men and Women*

	Men (%)	Women (%)
Essential fat	0–5	0–8
Optimal health	10–25	18–30
Optimal fitness	12–18	16–25
Athletes	5–13	12–22
Obesity	Above 25	Above 30

*A certain amount of fat in the body is essential for health, and optimal health can be achieved within quite a large range of percentages of body fat. Within that range are individuals in good physical condition, though not necessarily athletes. Individuals at both ends of the spectrum—either minimum body fat or a high proportion of fat—are at health risk.

Source: *The Physician and Sportsmedicine,* April 1986.

Experiments are being conducted with methods to measure body fat indirectly. One, called total body impedance, uses harmless, painless electric current to measure electrical resistance, which is related to the amount of body water, body density, and body fat. Unfortunately, the electrical resistance meters that claim to measure body fat are not very accurate. That's because measurements are through the feet exclusively, and such impedance measurements simply cannot assess the entire body.

The ideal percentage of body fat for men and women is shown in Table 2.2. If you have an opportunity to be tested, we recommend that you do so. But for most people concerned about weight, a look in the mirror will tell if the percentage of body fat—and body weight—is too high.

Increasingly, physicians, dietitians, and other health professionals are viewing weight in terms of the body mass index (BMI), a measure of body fat that corrects for height. It is derived by dividing weight in kilograms by the square of height in meters. The critical dividing line between healthy and unhealthy weight seems to be a BMI of 27. (Even better is a BMI of 25.) Beyond that point, the risk of heart disease, diabetes, and hypertension climbs rapidly.

Here's How to Determine Your Own BMI

First calculate your weight in kilograms by dividing pounds by 2.2. For example, a person weighing 150 pounds will have a weight in kilograms of 68. Next, calculate your height in meters by finding total inches. A person who is 6 feet tall is, by multiplying by 12 inches, 72 inches. A 5-foot tall person is 60 inches tall. Then multiply those inches by 2.50, since there are 2.50 centimeters per inch. Our six-footer would be 180 centimeters tall, while the five-footer would be 150 centimeters tall. There are 100 centimeters per meter, so the next step is to divide centimeters by 100. In our examples, the six-footer will be 1.8 meters tall, and our five-footer will be 1.5 meters tall. Finally, square the measurement in meters by multiplying it by itself, then divide weight in kilograms by that result. Thus, by this calculation, our six-footer would have a BMI of 68 ÷ 3.24 (the 3.24 is determined by multiplying 1.8 times 1.8), or a BMI of 20.9. A five-footer with the same weight would have a BMI of 30.2.

By these calculations a 6-foot-tall person weighing 150 pounds with a BMI of 20.9 would be well within the healthy zone. The same weight for the 5-foot-tall individual would result in a BMI of 30.2, significantly higher than desired and out of the healthful range. Needless to say, it's more practical for the five-footer to lose those extra pounds than to grow another foot in height. Here's a quick and easy way—without the problems of metric conversion—to determine your own BMI. Just plug your own numbers into this equation:

$$BMI = \frac{703 \times weight\ in\ pounds}{(height\ in\ inches)^2}$$

Here's an example for a person weighing 162 pounds at 5 feet 9 inches (69 inches):

$$BMI = \frac{703 \times 162}{69 \times 69}$$

$$BMI = \frac{113,886}{4761}$$

$$BMI = 24$$

Table 2.3 Body Mass Index (BMI)

Height	Weight				
5′1″	127	132	137	143	158
5′2″	131	136	142	147	164
5′3″	135	141	146	152	169
5′4″	140	145	151	157	174
5′5″	144	150	156	162	180
5′6″	148	150	156	162	186
5′7″	153	159	166	172	191
5′8″	158	164	171	177	197
5′9″	162	169	176	182	203
5′10″	167	174	181	188	207
5′11″	172	179	186	193	215
6′0″	177	184	191	199	221
6′1″	182	189	197	204	227
BMI	24*	25**	26**	27**	30***

*BMI of 24 or under: healthy
**BMI of 25–29: overweight
***BMI of 30 or more: extremely obese

With a BMI of 24, our example would be deemed healthy by National Heart, Lung, and Body Institute (NHLBI) guidelines. If he or she were to gain 7 pounds, however, the BMI would rise to 25, the cutoff point for being overweight. In the past, overweight was considered a BMI of 27 or greater. Those with a BMI of 30 or more are diagnosed as being clinically obese, requiring definite action to lose weight. Take a look at Table 2.3 to see how you do.

> **Y**ou must reach your goal weight to ensure permanent weight loss.

We strongly believe that it is important to establish a definite goal weight early in your weight loss efforts. As we've discovered, it's difficult to determine exactly what that goal weight should be, but the goal must be realistic. There are the factors of frame size and body fat percentage, and it may not be reasonable to expect an ultrathin appearance.

For many people there is a distinct time when weight began to pile on. If you have not always been as overweight as you are now, try to remember the time when you were most content with your size. Perhaps you were at what you consider an ideal weight in college or in the military or before your first child was born. After that time, for whatever reason, you began to gain weight, you fell into the metabolic trap of insulin resistance, and the weight seemed to come faster. Go through some early photographs to see the person you once were and could and will be again. That's your goal weight. Men and women who achieve their goal weights are more likely to keep the weight off permanently.

To see why, let's take the example of Laura, who came to the office at 250 pounds. At 5 feet 7 inches tall, she felt she should weigh 140, the weight she enjoyed in college. Laura responded beautifully to the diet program, and the pounds started coming off on schedule. Needless to say, Laura was pleased with her progress. Then at 160 pounds she decided that she had lost enough weight. Her friends and relatives were all telling her how skinny she looked. Some even urged her to gain some of her weight back. Soon the goal weight was forgotten. Surely a weight loss of 90 pounds was enough. But, since she wasn't exactly at goal weight, Laura didn't mind too much when she gained a few pounds. There was a party here, a nibble there, and before long she had gained much of her weight back.

Kathy, on the other hand, attained her goal of 130 pounds, a full 100-pound weight loss. Just as Laura had done, Kathy responded well to the program, but Kathy remained determined to meet her goal and did so in a reasonable amount of time. She then went through a stabilization period and ultimately into a maintenance program. She learned to add calories to her diet slowly until she neither gained nor lost weight. To our knowledge, Kathy remains at her desired 130 pounds.

Why is this matter of goal weight so important? There are both medical and psychological explanations. In medical terms Laura was still in the metabolic trap of insulin resistance. She never got out of it. By retaining some of her excessive body fat, along with salt and fluid, Laura didn't have a chance. She teetered on the brink of weight gain from the very beginning. Moreover, she never learned the skills to maintain weight.

On a psychological basis Laura was similarly in a danger zone. Compare her with the person who attempts to stop the cigarette habit by cutting back from two packs a day to three or four cigarettes. The habit is never broken. Such a person is constantly in a state of withdrawal, an uncomfortable feeling as anyone who has quit will testify. It is a rare person who can go from being an addicted smoker to having a few cigarettes daily. It's best to quit completely.

Similarly, Laura was not completely committed to the weight loss program. Since she already had some extra pounds over ideal, a few more didn't seem to make much difference. The goal weight was a future concept. She could always achieve her goal a few days or a few weeks later; she could always lose a few pounds tomorrow. But then there was another pound and then another few pounds—just like the person who smokes just one more cigarette. No wonder, then, that Laura failed in her ultimate effort. Kathy, having made the goal weight a reality, had a feeling of pride and achievement; she had something at stake.

Let's take our comparison with cigarette smoking further. Most former smokers will tell you, "Once a smoker, always a smoker." Those committed to staying away from tobacco will never take even one cigarette, realizing that if they smoke one cigarette, they will be hooked again. But on the brighter side, the longer one stays away from the cigarettes, the easier it gets. The moments of desperately wanting a smoke grow shorter and fewer. The smoker learns to not smoke. The overweight person learns to not eat what he or she knows he or she shouldn't eat. It's all part of the process of reaching your ideal weight.

About twenty years ago, public health authorities published leading articles emphasizing that obesity and its major consequences were urging physicians to view obesity as a disease entity to be diagnosed and treated with equal fervor to, say, cholesterol or blood pressure control. It's not enough for doctors to merely say, "You really ought to lose a few pounds," and to pass out a couple of pamphlets. Why all that emphasis? The medical community in general was trying to finally get the attention of the American public that weight was killing us, just as it continues to do so today.

Chapter 3

WHY THIS PROGRAM WORKS

This program is a terrific combination of education and good nutrition. It is this combination that can and will make a difference. A difference for life. It is wonderful to be in control again.
—L.J., LANSING, MICHIGAN

We have no record of the first case of obesity, but we can guess that it occurred when food was plentiful for the first time and people were able to rest more than they exercised. We also have no record of the first attempt to lose weight, but we certainly have a lot of material in more recent times.

The weight loss industry is a multimillion-dollar business. Weight loss centers, clinics, spas, and support groups flourish. Issue after issue, the covers of magazines announce the newest weight loss "breakthrough." Supermarket and pharmacy shelves are lined with pills, tablets, and other nostrums claiming to be magic potions. Late-night television offers mail-order miracles. People go from one weight loss fad to another, convinced that the new gimmick or the new book will finally work, even though all the ones before have failed. So perpetually hopeful are these people that the sale of weight loss mailing lists in and of itself is big business.

Yet with all this preoccupation with weight loss, and with all the highly touted solutions to this perplexing problem, overweight continues to plague the population. In fact, the number of

> **N**ever before has the U.S. population been so obese.

men and women who are significantly overweight grows annually. Why don't these diets work? Why can't someone come up with the way out of this continuing predicament?

There is no one, simple answer to these questions. But there are definite reasons why the pursuit of weight loss has so often been a difficult, if not futile, endeavor.

People tend to be taken in more easily by diets that promise much, especially those that give fast initial results. However, weight maintenance rather than weight loss is the more important consideration, since although many diets can produce at least some weight loss, the lost pounds tend to be regained. In fact, quite often more pounds are put on than were lost in the first place. So, when looking at the reasons why diets fail, we'll examine both weight loss and maintenance.

The difficulty with plans that virtually exclude food for a period of time, such as liquid protein diets and temporary fasting, is that the dieters never learn to handle foods in a normal way. At some point currently overweight men and women began to lose control over their eating patterns. Simply keeping them away from food doesn't teach them what they were doing wrong or how to change their habits. Many studies have shown, and our own work bears out, that in order to maintain weight loss, one must make some lifestyle changes. These changes call for both nutrition education and behavior modification.

Knowing the fundamentals of nutrition as they apply to eating habits is crucial to lasting weight loss, yet many dieters are inadequately informed about them. Ironically, many people who are overweight are nonetheless poorly nourished. When one begins to learn about how to choose foods wisely for their nutrient contributions, one is able to enjoy a wide variety of foods while still maintaining weight.

Behavior modification is integral to any weight loss plan. It can be simply adopting helpful strategies such as not eating while engaged in other activities such as watching television. But behavior modification is far more meaningful when it comes from examining not only habits but also attitudes. Self-image is a significant factor that can make or break one's commitment to weight loss. Any weight loss program that doesn't implement some aspect of behavior modification is unlikely to succeed. Throughout this book we offer advice and support from years of patient contact, to help implement the lifestyle changes that can really make a difference.

Many of the most popular diets involve unnatural eating patterns. Diets that have not been properly designed can pose some physical and mental problems. If a diet stresses a single food, it's unlikely one will be able to stay with it for the rest of one's life. How long can you stand to eat quantities of grapefruit every day? No matter how delectable any food is the first day, by the end of a month you might turn green just looking at it. Such a diet, if it does achieve weight loss, is doomed to fail in keeping that weight off.

The same holds true for diets that stress any one food category. Some of these diets make some absurd claims that combinations of foods are more or less "fattening" than the foods eaten alone or eaten in a given order. They claim that the body can't digest more than one food at a time. This is nonsense. The body's various digestive chemicals are quite capable of digesting different foods at once.

When any one type of food is stressed and others are eliminated on a permanent basis, there is the danger of malnutrition and other health threats. A number of books prescribe eating huge volumes of fruit, often to the exclusion of other foods. Such a diet may lead to severe diarrhea, occasionally to the extent that hospitalization is required to combat dehydration. Irritation of the digestive tract can prevent absorption of needed nutrients. Diets that eliminate bulk-forming foods on a permanent basis can cause constipation, not a trivial matter that can be eased by simply taking a laxative. We know today that inactivity of the colon is a risk factor for developing cancer.

Ultimately, even if some weight loss does occur temporarily from poorly planned diet programs, weight regain will occur when it becomes either physically or mentally impossible to continue to follow such limited regimens.

In the 1950s and 1960s, dieting that used drugs came into vogue as doctors frequently wrote prescriptions for amphetamines to depress the appetite, reducing calorie intake. While the drugs often worked, they fostered dependency and adverse reactions including jitteriness, irritability, and sleeplessness. All too often other drugs were prescribed to counteract those reactions. This practice, referred to in the medical community as "rainbow therapy" for the many colors of the pills and tablets, is much less prevalent today.

The manufacture of amphetamines has been greatly curtailed, but there are a number of over-the-counter nostrums that have the same, though milder, effects.

The once popular drug combination known as "fen-phen" (fenfluramine and phentermine) has been removed from the market along with Redux (dexfenfluramine) because of the potential to develop primary pulmonary hypertension as well as problems with heart valves.

Given the drawbacks, danger, and ineffectiveness of the methods of weight control described thus far, most nutritionists and physicians have relied for years on the oldest weight loss advice we know of—cut back on total calories.

As a general rule, weight gain is the result of consuming too many and expending too few calories—eating too much and exercising too little. Genetics also plays an important role. Some people are more predisposed to being overweight than others. Some people gain weight more easily than others, needing fewer calories to put on extra pounds. But everyone, regardless of family history, will gain weight by eating too much and exercising too little.

Dietitians, then, commonly recommend diets that provide needed nutrients without unnecessary calories—usually a 1,200- to 1,500-calorie diet based on a variety of foods. For many people, especially for those with only 5 to 15 pounds to lose, this is all it takes. But these diets don't work for everyone; they have distinct limitations.

For one thing, not all foods work in the same way in terms of weight gain. It has been found that carbohydrates and protein provide 4 calories per gram, fat supplies 9, and alcohol 7. Moreover, the body doesn't self-limit fat intake in the same way it limits the intake of other foods. You never hear about someone gorging on fruit, for example, even after having eaten a quantity sufficient to suppress hunger. We have an apparently unlimited ability or tendency to consume fat. The body has a shut-off mechanism for both protein and carbohydrate, but not for fat.

Even supposing that merely reducing total calories could be effective regardless of circumstances and the type of food eaten, for the person with 50, 70, or 100 pounds to lose, it would take an inordinately long period of time for such a regimen to be completely effective. Furthermore, during that entire period of time, the dieter is bound to experience pangs of hunger regularly, and few people are willing to be hungry every day for months or even a year or more.

Another reason the simple "eat less" approach doesn't always work is that an important part of any successful weight loss program is exercise. It used to be thought that exercise was beneficial simply because it burns calories. We now know there's more to exercise than that. In addition to burning calories at the time of exertion, it increases the metabolic rate at which calories are utilized for some time after exertion. Exercise also increases one's sense of well-being and ability to relax. It builds muscle tissue, which, in turn, burns calories. That helps to explain why people with more lean muscle tend to have less of a weight problem. Exercise during weight loss inhibits the loss of muscle tissue, allowing the body to keep the lean and lose the fat. And finally, it plays the crucial role of regulating insulin levels. (Exercise is discussed in Chapter 7.)

Even the combination of calorie reduction and exercise is often ineffective, particularly with significantly overweight men and women, and as the degree of obesity increases, so does the failure rate of dieting.

When Dr. Atkins published his *Diet Revolution*, he advocated strict avoidance of carbohydrates but allowed all the meat and fat one wanted to eat. Because the diet worked, and people lost weight as promised, this approach became popular. But the diet had a number of flaws. Dieters' cholesterol levels rose significantly, increasing the risk of heart disease. When dieters returned to their former eating habits, they quickly regained the lost weight because no provision was made for exercise, inadequate advice was provided about future behavioral changes, and no information was given about the causes of the initial obesity, how the diet worked, and why a return to old eating habits would cause the weight to be regained.

Commercial weight loss companies developed programs that are based on natural foods, limit fat and carbohydrate, provide sufficient protein, include vitamin and mineral supplements, and recommend getting physician permission to follow the diet. Some clinics and spas use nurses and nutritionists to supervise progress.

Many of the commercial operations have the right idea. They call for mild exercise on a daily basis. Clients follow a diet of 600 to 1,000 calories, which allows for a satisfying rate of weight loss. Limiting carbohydrates leads to a mild state of ketosis, which diminishes hunger. Guidance in behavior modification improves future eating habits. And tips provided by supervising nurses and nutritionists supply the support that dieters need.

These programs work, but clients never learn that obesity has an underlying neuroendocrine cause. That's because when these programs were designed that cause had not yet been identified. More-over, these programs come with a high price tag not everyone can afford.

During all the years of diet experimentation, researchers have looked at the relationships among obesity, diabetes, and insulin. Numerous medical publications have shown that obese and diabetic individuals are extremely unresponsive to insulin. Certain foods trigger the release of large amounts of the hormone, but the body does not utilize it properly. Obese individuals usually show abnormally high insulin levels in the blood. And high levels of insulin lead to storage rather than usage of fats as well as to sodium and fluid retention.

Recently we've learned that hyperinsulinism may also be a culprit in coronary heart disease. Insulin stimulates the body's production of an enzyme that causes the liver to produce cholesterol. Oversupply of insulin in the blood may also stimulate changes in the arterial walls that promote formation of fatty plaques, which are involved in coronary heart disease. Insulin resistance may explain why Type 2 diabetics are four times as likely as nondiabetics to develop heart disease.

The result is that a person who has been significantly overweight for a prolonged period of time is no longer capable of losing weight by adhering to a program of decreased caloric intake and increased exercise that would work for other people. His or her body functions to maintain its weight. It makes sense, then, that an effective dietary approach must consider the role of insulin in overweight and must provide patients with an understanding of how insulin works and how to control it.

> The condition of hyperinsulinism is known as the meta-bolic trap.

The protein-sparing modified-fast diet does, indeed, control insulin levels in the blood, allowing for the burning of stored fats and the release of previously retained fluids. I used this approach in treating obese patients in my practice, often those who were originally referred for other endocrine disorders.

This diet is not essential for everyone. As stated earlier, those who have just a few pounds to lose will probably succeed by simply limiting the number of calories, especially fat calories, in the diet and by increasing the amount of exercise. However, everyone can benefit from information on endocrine function, behavior modification, exercise, support techniques, and procedures to assure stabilization and maintenance of weight loss. All of this information is included in the following chapters.

The Insulin Control Diet program is designed for men and women at least 20 percent over their ideal body weights. It provides a way to reverse the process of hyperinsulinism so that your body can switch gears, start to burn excess fat as fuel, supply your brain with the calming neurotransmitter serotonin so you'll sleep well at night and be relaxed during the day, eliminate stored salt and water, improve your energy level, and bring your metabolism back to normal. This diet program ensures enduring weight loss of 2 to 3 pounds per week for women and 3 to 4 pounds for men, without much hunger. It includes an easy, enjoyable exercise regimen. It provides information on sleep enhancement, behavior modification, nutrition, and the underlying causes of obesity.

If our promise sounds just as exaggerated as those made by countless weight loss charlatans, we ask only that you stick with it. Our approach is based on proven scientific facts, with case histories to back them up. Within a reasonable amount of time you will have shed excess pounds and inches, and you will be able to show your friends and relatives that *this* diet works.

> The Insulin Control Diet ensures satisfying weight loss of up to 3 pounds per week for women and 4 pounds for men, without much hunger.

This program offers a medical solution to a medical problem. It is not to be taken lightly. It is safe and effective only when used under the supervision of your physician. It is not meant for use by those with Type 1, insulin-dependent diabetes. There are certain contraindications to following this strenuous approach to weight loss: kidney and liver disorders, recent heart attack, and pregnancy and lactation. We intend the book to be a bridge between doctor and patient, a way for both to work together in order to slash the considerable health risk posed by overweight.

The first step is to schedule an appointment with your doctor. Discuss this book and your desire to follow the diet. Make photocopies of this chapter and of "Doctor to Doctor," which appears just before Chapter 1. Show these pages to your physician so he or she will understand the program's rationale and approach. As time goes on, he or she may wish to read the rest of the book as well.

Next, schedule regular appointments. Your doctor may want to see you every two, three, or four weeks. Most of your questions will be answered in the following pages, but during these appointments your physician will be able to address specific, individual problems and concerns.

Guidance and support, designed to increase commitment and motivation, are contained in Chapter 10. Take a look at it right after you complete this chapter to get an overview and a few tips you can put into effect immediately. Then read it again as you follow the program, paying particular attention to one strategy each day.

Next, start keeping a diet diary (see the example that follows). Use a bound notebook rather than loose pages. Every time you eat or drink anything, record the type and amount of food in the diary. Most people don't realize what and how much they eat. By recording everything you eat and drink, you'll become aware of your true food intake. That information will be helpful in making appropriate changes. Also record where and when you eat and any unusual feelings or reactions to your circumstances immediately before and after eating. We can't stress the value of this diary too much, and we'll refer to it from time to time in the coming pages.

We'll be discussing some of the benefits of weight loss in detail, but only you know how important it is to you to lose the weight that you've come to hate and that threatens your well-being. Anything that important is worth working for, and this program does take more than a little effort. But as the days and weeks go by, we're confident that you'll agree it's worth it!

So, get started right away. Don't put it off a day more. Here's your agenda:

- Make an appointment to see your physician.
- Read Chapter 10 on support to help your motivation.
- Make photocopies of this chapter and "Doctor to Doctor" to take to your physician.
- Start a diet diary today, recording everything you eat and drink.
- Read the balance of this book.

Diet Diary

Eating Log Week _____ , from _____ to _____

Week's Weight Loss: _____ Current Weight: _____

Breakfast	Breakfast	Breakfast	Breakfast	Breakfast	Breakfast	Breakfast
Lunch	Lunch	Lunch	Lunch	Lunch	Lunch	Lunch
Dinner	Dinner	Dinner	Dinner	Dinner	Dinner	Dinner
Snacks	Snacks	Snacks	Snacks	Snacks	Snacks	Snacks
Total carbs:	Total carbs:	Total carbs:	Total carbs:	Total carbs:	Total carbs:	Total carbs:
Ketosis: AM PM	Ketosis: AM PM	Ketosis: AM PM	Ketosis: AM PM	Ketosis: AM PM	Ketosis: AM PM	Ketosis: AM PM
Strong cravings yes no Energy up down	Strong cravings yes no Energy up down	Strong cravings yes no Energy up down	Strong cravings yes no Energy up down	Strong cravings yes no Energy up down	Strong cravings yes no Energy up down	Strong cravings yes no Energy up down

Chapter 4

YOUR PERSONAL ENDOCRINE SYSTEM

I think the turning point for me was when I finally understood the link between sleep, carbohydrate intake, and insulin production. When you understand the mechanics of a theory it makes it so much easier to put that theory into practice. I now understand how increased carbohydrate intake throws the body into the vicious cycle of increased blood sugar and insulin production, and the weight gain that ultimately follows. This knowledge helps me make more intelligent food choices. It's a program I will rely on for the rest of my life.
—P.L., DES PLAINES, ILLINOIS

The body has a number of regulatory systems that keep it in a state of physiological balance. We can ski on snowy slopes or lie on a sunny beach, yet our internal temperature remains at 98.6°F. We can drink copious amounts of liquids one day and almost none the next, yet the amount of fluids within our tissues stays fairly constant. The tendency of the body to keep everything in a steady state is referred to as homeostasis, which, literally translated from the Greek, is "same standing."

Our bodies attempt to regulate our weights from the time of maturity, but we challenge our control systems by eating too much and exercising too little. Even with such challenges, many of us maintain or can maintain approximately the same weight from our late teens or early twenties on through middle and old age. Even if we gain weight after a period of overeating, most of us can, with a degree of desire and commitment, shed the extra pounds and keep them off. However, some of us appear unable to control and maintain weight despite the best of intentions and efforts.

In order to understand such a system failure and to grasp the methods by which the Insulin Control Diet works so well, we need to examine our bodies' regulatory systems, focusing on the two major control centers—the nervous system and two categories of glands.

The nervous system can be compared with a network of electrical wires interconnected with a main power source. The nerves travel throughout the body from their origins in the brain and spinal cord. They communicate information to the brain, which, in turn, sends signals to various parts of the body to perform a given action. The action may be voluntary or involuntary. Unlike connected wires, however, the nerves are not directly attached. There are spaces, called synapses, between one nerve sending a signal and another one receiving it. These spaces are filled by chemical substances, called neurotransmitters, which function in a variety of ways both to facilitate nervous impulses and to affect our state of mind.

One such neurotransmitter is serotonin. This chemical regulator, produced from the amino acid tryptophan, helps to keep us calm and relaxed. Without enough of it we feel irritable and depressed and are unable to sleep well. You may know those feelings well, as they are often associated with the metabolic trap of hyperinsulinism.

Glands are groups of cells that produce and secrete substances for a variety of uses. Two types of glands are exocrine and endocrine. Exocrine glands secrete their chemical products into ducts that conduct them to where they are needed. For example, salivary glands produce saliva, which is transported through ducts to the mouth. Similarly, the pancreas produces digestive enzymes that enter the intestine by way of ducts.

Endocrine glands have no such ducts and secrete their chemical products into the bloodstream. To facilitate the transfer of product into the bloodstream, each endocrine gland has an abundant network of tiny blood vessels, or capillaries. The substances secreted by the endocrine glands are called hormones. The way exocrine secretions such as digestive enzymes affect nutrition are rather obvious.

The effects of the endocrine glands are not always so clear, and some work in ways that were previously misunderstood.

Not all of the endocrine glands influence digestion, nutrition, and weight regulation. The principal ductless glands that do are the pituitary at the base of the brain, the thyroid in the neck, the islets of Langerhans in the pancreas, in the abdomen, the adrenals next to the kidneys, and the gonads in the pelvic cavity (female ovaries) or the scrotum (male testes). We will consider only briefly the parathyroid glands, also found in the neck, which have little direct influence on metabolism and nutrition.

PITUITARY

The pituitary gland sits in a well-protected cavity at the base of the skull behind the eyes and between the ears. Although it is only as large as the tip of the little finger, the pituitary gland produces at least eight hormones that directly affect the body and that control the functions of other glands. Because other endocrine glands are to one degree or another governed by the pituitary, it is often called the master gland.

The thyroid, adrenals, and gonads are regulated by hormones secreted by the anterior lobe of the pituitary. These are called trophic, supporting, or stimulating hormones because they trigger the production and release of other hormones in the target glands. In addition to these supporting hormones, the anterior pituitary produces growth hormone, which is responsible for skeletal growth; prolactin, which stimulates breast milk production and favors the storage of body fat; and melanocyte-stimulating hormone, which increases the production of melanin, a skin pigment. Melanocyte-stimulating hormone is derived from the larger precursor of adrenocorticotrophic hormone (ACTH). The precursor is called *proopiomelanocorticotrophin* because it also provides opioids—endorphins and encephalins.

The posterior portion of the pituitary stores two hormones produced in the hypothalamus, a nearby portion of the brain. Oxytocin stimulates contractions of the womb during labor and helps milk letdown in lactation. Antidiuretic hormone causes kidneys to remove water from urine as it is formed, decreasing urine volume.

ADRENALS

There are two adrenal glands, one located above each kidney. Each gland is divided into two segments, the outer cortex and the inner medulla. The cortex secretes three groups of hormones. Glucocorticoids maintain energy and well-being and tend to raise levels of blood sugar by blocking the action of insulin. Mineralocorticoids regulate sodium and potassium concentration and fluid homeostasis, thus affecting water retention and blood pressure. The gonadocorticoids, or sex hormones (estrogens and androgens), have little influence on nutrition and digestion, but they do affect the percentage and location of body fat.

The adrenal medulla synthesizes adrenaline and noradrenaline, also known as epinephrine and norepinephrine. These are the hormones involved in the "fight or flight" response to danger. We've all experienced the feelings these hormones engender when we are frightened, threatened, or excited. These hormones depress appetite, stimulate metabolism, and increase blood pressure.

GONADS

The gonads, or sex glands, are under complicated control, largely by way of the pituitary gland and its trophic hormones. In the female the gonadotropic hormones and the hormones produced in the ovaries and placenta regulate the menstrual cycle, maintain pregnancy, and stimulate lactation. Follicle-stimulating hormone stimulates the ovary to ripen an egg-carrying cavity called the follicle. When the follicle is ripe and the egg is ready to be released, luteinizing hormone acts to stimulate ovulation, or the release of the egg into the fallopian tube. The corpus luteum (yellow body), which produces progesterone, is then formed from the collapsed follicle. Progesterone makes the uterus more receptive to the fertilized egg.

The estrogens, a group of closely related female sex hormones, are produced in the follicle as well as in the adrenal cortex. They are responsible for the development and maintenance of secondary sex characteristics, including breast development and deposition of adipose tissue or fat in strategic areas of the body. Because of the action of the estrogens there is a higher percentage of fat in the bodies of females. While an athletically slender male's total weight will be from 12 to 15 percent fat, that of a similarly athletic and slender female will be about 20 percent.

Hormonal control is not as complicated in the male. Testes make testosterone, the most important male hormone, in cells outside the sperm factory. Luteinizing hormone, sometimes called interstitial cell–stimulating hormone, stimulates the testosterone-producing cells. Follicle-stimulating hormone and testosterone interact to promote sperm production.

THYROID

The thyroid is the most misrepresented of all the glands. It does in fact help to control the body's metabolic rate, but the often-heard claim that obesity can be traced to an underactive thyroid gland is seldom if ever true.

Located in front of the windpipe, or trachea, in the throat, the thyroid gland weighs less than an ounce in normal individuals. Within its tissues it combines iodine obtained from the diet with the amino acid tyrosine to form the hormone thyroxine (T4). But before the thyroid can exert its influence, thyroxine must be converted to the more active form of triiodothyronine (T3). T3 regulates the various enzymes that control energy metabolism and thus influence all metabolic processes. The effects of an overactive or underactive thyroid gland can be dramatic.

Both T4 and T3 are under the influence of the pituitary gland by way of thyroid-stimulating hormone (TSH). When levels of thyroid hormone in the blood fall, TSH rises, causing the production and release into the blood of both T4 and T3. Increases in T4 and T3 levels signal the pituitary to stop releasing TSH. This is known as "negative feedback." Analogous to a thermostat, which turns off heat at a certain level, this mechanism has been sometimes called the "thyrostat." The most accurate way to determine if the thyroid is functioning normally is to measure the level of TSH in the blood. Even the slightest drop in thyroid hormone will increase TSH levels.

When the thyroid gland produces inadequate amounts of hormone over a long time, the person may become tired easily, have dry skin, and feel cold, even in rooms where others are comfortable. But in documented cases of such prolonged hypothyroidism (underactive thyroid), there rarely is weight gain of more than 15 or 20 pounds. That gain is mainly due to the accumulation of mucinous tissue, a gelatinous material that absorbs water. Patients with hypothyroidism seldom if ever gain substantial amounts of adipose tissue. On the other hand, hyperthyroidism (overactive thyroid) will usually result in some weight loss. There is no evidence to substantiate the idea that an underactive thyroid has anything to do with obesity.

There are some people with elevated TSH without symptoms of hypothyroidism for whom thyroid hormone administration is indicated. But for people with normal TSH, thyroid hormone administration will not in any way benefit them and may lead to significant side effects. Inappropriate administration of excess thyroid medication runs the risks of inducing cardiac arrhythmias and aggravating osteoporosis.

PARATHYROIDS

There are usually four rice-grain-sized parathyroid glands found in the neck just outside the thyroid gland. They produce parathyroid hormone, the chief regulator of calcium balance in the body. Their major nutritional connection is with vitamin D, which is used to treat the low calcium state caused by parathyroid deficiency.

PANCREAS

While the role of the thyroid gland in weight gain and loss has been exaggerated, the important influence of insulin, the major hormone of the pancreas, has long been recognized. Insulin is one of the hormones produced by the endocrine pancreas, the other being glucagon.

The pancreas produces two types of secretions. Digestive enzymes (exocrine secretions), delivered to the gut through the pancreatic duct, are produced by masses of cells called acini. Hormones (endocrine secretions) are manufactured in the portion of the gland called the islets of Langerhans. The islets contain two major types of cells. The beta cells produce insulin, and the alpha cells make glucagon.

The two hormones have opposing effects and work in a system of checks and balances.

THE FUNCTIONS OF INSULIN

Most people have heard of insulin because of its role in diabetes. For centuries physicians recognized the disease as characterized by sugar in the urine, but little was known of what caused it and how to treat it. The diagnosis of diabetes in children was a death warrant until 1921, when Frederick Banting and Charles Best isolated insulin from the pancreas and demonstrated that it could reduce blood sugar levels when given by injection.

We now more fully understand insulin's role in metabolism. The hormone acts as a kind of spark plug to the mechanism that allows glucose (blood sugar) in the blood to enter the cell, where it can be used for energy. Without insulin, sugar builds up in the blood to dangerous and even life-threatening levels. There are two main types of diabetes. In Type 1, or insulin-dependent, diabetes the pancreas does not produce insulin or does so at inadequate levels. Thus insulin must be supplied by injection. Type 1 diabetes most typically occurs in the early years and so was previously called childhood, or juvenile-onset, diabetes. In Type 2, or noninsulin-dependent, diabetes the pancreas produces sufficient insulin, but the body does not use it efficiently, allowing blood sugar levels to rise. Type 2 diabetes is usually manifested in middle age and so was called maturity-onset diabetes.

Because of the essential role of insulin in the body's metabolism and its life-saving aspects for diabetics, most people view insulin in only the most positive light. But insulin has a number of functions other than allowing the cell to use glucose from the blood, some of which can have a negative impact on weight control and general health.

After you eat a meal, the pancreas secretes mainly insulin into the bloodstream to maintain an optimal blood sugar level. However, other hormones, chiefly glucagon, but also adrenaline, cortisol, and growth hormone, act against insulin to prevent the blood sugar from dropping too low. The supply of glucose is essential not only for the body's physical energy but also for brain function and survival of sensitive nervous tissue.

When there isn't sufficient food-derived glucose in the blood for the brain's fuel, the body produces its own, at first through the breakdown of stored glycogen, or animal starch, in the liver and then through a process called gluconeogenesis, literally, the production of new glucose. In gluconeogenesis amino acids are converted to glucose. If amino acids are available as part of the food supply, the body will use them for this purpose. If not, protein from muscle tissue will be broken down to provide amino acids.

Gluconeogenesis, which is inhibited by insulin and promoted by glucagon, is a natural bodily process and may be implemented at times between meals. It is the body's way to attempt to stave off starvation by quite literally feeding the brain from the body's own muscle tissue.

An alternative source of brain fuel the body can use is ketones, which can be formed from liberated fatty acids stored in adipose tissue. Ketones can supply energy as efficiently as glucose can, and the body will contentedly utilize them for long periods with no adverse reactions. After an extended period of starvation or carbohydrate restriction, ketones are formed by the body to supplement glucose derived from gluconeogenesis when there is not enough insulin in the blood to prevent their formation. Ketogenesis requires the influence of glucagon to proceed. The delicate balance between insulin and glucagon is critical in this regard. In a normally functioning body new glucose will be formed during the night when the person sleeps, when insulin levels are down and glucagon levels rise. Also, at such times fatty acids are readily liberated from adipose tissue and converted into fuel, just as nature intended. During states of obesity this process can be frustrated by the abnormally high levels of insulin that persist in the blood.

Gluconeogenesis and ketogenesis are then two processes affected by insulin in addition to glucose utilization. Insulin has still other complicated actions that affect many parts of the body. Insulin is involved with the disposal of amino acids, fatty acids, and electrolytes. It causes a buildup of triglycerides, the storage form of fatty acids, and it inhibits their release from fat cells. Insulin also increases the formation of cholesterol in the liver and similar steroid hormones in the adrenals and sex glands. It favors protein buildup and storage, and it increases the formation of liver and muscle glycogen, the only form of stored carbohydrate available for supplementary energy production. Since insulin favors salt and water retention, it can aggravate hypertension. It also increases the activity of the sympathetic nervous system, which can raise blood pressure.

In total, when insulin levels are high in the blood, a number of negative things can and do occur. In people who have become obese, sometimes even those who are only 25 or 30 pounds overweight, insulin levels remain high, the efficiency of the hormone in facilitating the passage of glucose into the cells is lessened, and more is required to maintain normal blood glucose levels. Insulin also is less able to minimize new glucose formation, another potential source of hyperglycemia, unless more insulin is provided. This is the state of insulin resistance that leads to hyperinsulinism.

Insulin Resistance

How do cells become insulin resistant? There may be a decrease in the number of the insulin receptors on the cell membrane that bind insulin and allow it to act. The insulin receptors may no longer respond to insulin as they should to let glucose enter the cell. There may be defects within the cell that interfere with glucose utilization. Research has found that in obesity, insulin resistance in muscle is not due to an abnormality of receptors that bind insulin but rather to the failure to activate enzymes that mobilize the glucose transport system within the cell.

There are four major causes for developing insulin resistance. First is obesity itself, which develops over time, and in which adipose (fat) tissue produces substances (adipokines) that move to muscle tissue to selectively block the blood sugar–lowering effect of insulin. The second cause is Type 2 diabetes, in which insulin resistance may precede diabetes and may or may not be associated with obesity. Third, when blood sugar levels exceed 300 mg/dL, or perhaps even less, the hyperglycemia can trigger insulin resistance. The fourth cause is stress, physical, emotional, or traumatic. It increases insulin-neutralizing stress hormones such as cortisol, adrenaline, and glucagon as well as growth hormone.

Because the blood sugar control by insulin is inefficient in some people, the body tries to compensate by making *more* insulin and levels begin to soar. The same phenomenon occurs in obese patients with Type 2 diabetes. There is usually more than enough insulin in the blood, but the body simply is not using it properly. In fact, administering more insulin by injection in order to lower blood sugar levels in such patients perpetuates the problem. The answer is diet, exercise, and good sleep to lower insulin requirements, not to give patients more of it. These measures are not adequate unless they are linked with improved sleep quality, provided by serotonin replenishment.

Even though sugar levels are elevated in the blood owing to the ineffectiveness of insulin to control it, the insulin continues to function normally in other respects. Thus the person lacking sufficient brain serotonin experiences carbohydrate (especially sugary food) cravings. As more carbohydrates are consumed, the body produces more insulin to attempt to deal with them. That additional insulin retains its ability to build fat, and thereby the insulin resistance factors (adipokines), contributing to the need for more insulin.

Without adequate glucose entering the cell for energy and with a reduced ability to utilize fatty acids stored for alternative energy, paired with inadequate sleep, it is little wonder that overweight men and women are tired and listless.

Now we have an overweight person, who cannot properly use glucose in the blood for cellular energy, who continues to store fatty acids in the tissues as increasing pounds of fat, and who is tired, irritable, and depressed. And he or she must now face yet another of insulin's adverse reactions. Part of this hormone's function is to store salt, which facilitates water retention. When insulin levels soar, salt and water storage increase to formidable proportions, and the person gains more weight. Also, the salt retention causes blood pressure to rise. Increased responsiveness to adrenaline aggravates the tendency to high blood pressure.

In this situation typical efforts at weight loss are frustrating. Diuretics are extremely dangerous and can cause a sufficient decrease in potassium to induce cardiac arrest. As energy levels drop and sleepless nights continue, it's not surprising that such individuals engage in little physical activity and frequently become lethargic and close to immobile. In the worst cases, inactivity is accompanied by feeding cravings for carbohydrates that can never be fully satisfied until its source, namely inadequate sleep, is corrected by serotonin replenishment.

Many an overweight person in this situation attempts to explain his or her feelings of powerlessness, but physicians, friends, and family respond by suggesting the problem is simply a lack of willpower. Yet this seemingly hopeless condition does have scientific foundation, as just explained. The overweight person is caught in an insidious metabolic trap.

KETOSIS

The key to unlocking the metabolic trap is the physiological process ketosis, in which the body's liver produces substances called ketones from fatty acids that have been stored as adipose tissue. Free fatty acids are normally liberated from stored triglycerides through exercise. However, because of hyperinsulinism free fatty acid mobilization is markedly but not totally impaired in obese subjects. On our low calorie, low carbohydrate weight loss diet, which reduces levels of circulating insulin, free fatty acid mobilization is improved. Fat thus becomes the major source of energy. The body begins to use its stored fat as fuel for the brain and energy for the body as a replacement for glucose.

To allow this process to occur, insulin production must be decreased and glucagon production must be increased. A substantial restriction of carbohydrate intake facilitates both. With less carbohydrate the body gradually slows down the excessive production of insulin and secretes more glucagon.

To reiterate and clarify the importance of this phenomenon, here's what happens when insulin production decreases:

1. The body can mobilize its stores of fatty acids to be used as fuel, rather than to be kept as adipose tissue.
2. Hunger and carbohydrate craving decline, especially with the added influence of increased serotonin from trazodone.
3. Salt retention and water retention decrease, allowing excess fluid to be excreted naturally, with concomitant weight loss.
4. Blood pressure falls due to loss of sodium and fluid and decreased effectiveness of adrenaline in constricting arterial walls.

Most patients report entering the state of mild ketosis needed to achieve weight loss within three days after beginning this program.

Testing for ketosis is easily done with KetoStix (manufactured by the Ames Company). The urine is collected in a container, a plastic stick is dipped into the sample, and fifteen seconds later the color of the stick is compared to a chart on the container. Many prefer to simply hold the KetoStix in the urine stream to moisten the tip of the strip. There's no need to soak the strip. Beige indicates negative ketosis, pink mild ketosis, purple moderate ketosis, and deeper purple significant ketosis.

With this program you can expect to see pink to light purple changes in the stick's color. The deepness of color will vary with the amount of fluid excreted in the urine. If you have consumed the recommended eight 8-ounce glasses of water daily, the urine will be quite diluted, and the color will not be into the deep purple range. Even mild ketosis signals lowered insulin production. When you see the stick change color to pink or light purple, you know your body is freeing itself from the metabolic trap.

In testing for ketones, ideally in the morning and at bedtime, you may see some fluctuation in color, simply because the urine may be more or less dilute, depending on the amount of fluid you have been consuming. The daily ritual of testing your urine will act as a motivator, a reminder, to follow the program.

The Dangers of Ketosis

Ketosis has been misunderstood by both the lay public and the medical profession. There is such a thing as good ketosis, a state that can be tolerated by the body for long periods of time, but we have to distinguish this mild, beneficial ketosis from the condition that can be produced by uncontrolled diets. Diets in which fat consumption is unlimited may induce more severe ketosis, with side effects including nausea, vomiting, and dehydration. In the Insulin Control Diet the only significant fat source is the stored adipose tissue of the dieter. As a result, at no time does the degree of ketosis produced exceed the tolerance of the body. If you follow the advice of this program, you will not be striving for a deep purple KetoStix reading, and you will never enter severe ketosis. Instead, you'll experience the rich, rewarding benefits of mild ketosis.

You should also not confuse this mild ketosis with keto-acidosis, a condition associated with uncontrolled diabetes. The balance between acidity and alkalinity of blood and body fluids is called *acid-base balance*. Normally it is maintained slightly on the alkaline side by adjustments made in the kidneys and lungs. Ketones are acidic and need to be balanced by appropriate adjustments to prevent an increase in the acidity of the body. In the severely uncontrolled diabetic, ketones are massively overproduced and overwhelm the body's adaptive mechanisms. In this state of acidosis, patients may proceed to coma and death. It is this association that makes some physicians fear ketosis of any sort, even if it may be beneficial. In our program the body can easily eliminate the ketones, the acid-base balance is maintained, and it is not possible to proceed to a state of acidosis.

Another criticism leveled against ketosis is that it can aggravate gout, a painful condition resulting from the buildup of uric acid in the blood. Critics point out that ketones and uric acid are excreted through the same pathway; thus heavy ketone production causes the uric acid to rise. If recommended fluid amounts are consumed, in most cases uric acid can be properly eliminated in the urine. It is true that in male patients with a tendency to high uric acid, ketosis could result in gout. However, your physician can prevent this by administering appropriate medication to lower uric acid levels, such as allopurinol.

Ketosis is an essential part of this weight loss program. As used in this program it is perfectly safe, and it is effective in unlocking the metabolic trap. Ketosis is the bridge that helps one return to a normal metabolic state.

The concept behind the Insulin Control Diet is well founded in scientific and medical fact. It has been tested and proven safe and effective in hundreds of patients. No serious problems have been noted, and none are expected to occur in individuals who follow the program with medical supervision.

Now you know about how your endocrine system works and the importance of good sleep in weight control. With that knowledge you are ready to unlock the metabolic trap.

Chapter 5

GOOD FOODS, GOOD MOODS

The pounds quickly vanished. I felt alert,
energetic, and satisfied by the food I ate.
There were absolutely no cravings. I fit
in all my clothes and am the thinnest
I've been in years. I feel fantastic and
owe it all to you!
—P.C., AMES, IOWA

There's no question that the foods we eat have much to do with the way we feel and the way we feel about ourselves. Various substances in food create bodily reactions that affect everyone's moods. And in overweight people who have fallen into the metabolic trap, their conditions and bodily reactions can increase the potential for depression and irritability. In addition, for many people being overweight engenders a sense of helplessness and hopelessness, especially regarding their desire to lose weight. They lose interest in things and activities around them. Many feel guilty about their weights, a feeling that our society aggravates at every turn by praising and rewarding the slender and condemning the overweight. Many overweight people become socially withdrawn. And the more overweight they become, the less welcoming our society seems.

Taken together, these aspects of the overweight person's mental state—helplessness, hopelessness, guilt, loss of interests, and social withdrawal—can collectively be termed depression. Many patients who have come to my office for help simply characterize themselves as depressed.

That depression is not solely a psychological condition that can be altered by a shift in attitude or circumstance. Depression associated with being overweight has its origins in physical phenomena. Trying to treat the psychological symptoms alone, whether by seeing a therapist or taking medications, usually does not meet with success.

Many overweight patients come to me either currently taking antidepressant drugs and tranquilizers or seeking them. Many expect that a prescription for this pill or that tablet will cure their problems—both of depression and overweight. Some patients are disappointed, at first, when the prescription pad for these drugs doesn't come out as expected. But almost all leave my office with an upbeat feeling. They've learned during that first visit there's a physical reason for their mood and a scientific basis for their persistent problems with weight—in short, that it isn't all their fault.

But we should clarify one thing at the start. When talking about depression, we must draw a line between the normal reactions of overweight men and women to their conditions and abnormal responses that would be defined as pathological. Almost everyone coming into the office suffers some degree of depression, although the symptoms may vary from person to person. *But*—and it's an important *but*—only a few patients are depressed to the point where life no longer seems worth living. I have encountered some patients who, when questioned even tentatively, volunteer that they are indeed desperate or are considering suicide.

If you feel that way, then by all means seek qualified medical or psychological assistance. Your depression may be partly a result of your weight problem, but likely it's a more deep-seated condition requiring professional help. Do you have frequent feelings that life is not worth living? Do you feel that there is never any joy in life and that waking up in the morning is the beginning of another day of misery? Have you increasingly shunned social contact? Have others commented more and more frequently about your mental state? If so, seek medical help right away. Take care of those problems, and then come back to this book and its program.

For most of you, the solutions in these pages will help to turn around negative feelings, as part of the process of freeing yourself from the metabolic trap.

NEUROTRANSMITTERS

Let's start with one of the most essential ingredients to living an active, enjoyable life: a good night's sleep. Many people who are seriously overweight have difficulty falling asleep, staying asleep, and waking with a rested feeling. Such sleep disorders, along with daytime feelings of irritability and anxiety, are an integral part of your total overweight problem, a part of the metabolic trap.

To understand this and to learn how to implement the solution, it is important to understand a bit about how your nervous system works. The brain is composed of billions of nerve cells called neurons, which are separated by gaps called synapses. To transmit a nerve impulse from one neuron to another and to communicate information throughout the nervous system, somehow those gaps must be bridged. This is done by way of chemicals known as neurotransmitters.

Today we know there are forty neurotransmitters. All are derived from amino acids, the building blocks of protein. There are twenty-two amino acids. Of those, eight cannot be produced by the body and must be consumed as part of our diet. They are called essential amino acids, meaning it is essential that we ingest them. (All the amino acids are necessary for life. Since the body can produce the other fourteen, they are called nonessential, meaning they are not essential parts of the diet.) Fortunately, unless one is on a particularly stringent diet, such as strict vegetarianism with absolutely no animal protein, getting enough of the essential amino acids isn't a problem.

Amino acids are sent to all parts of the body through the bloodstream. Those we are concerned with in reference to mood problems are the ones going to the brain. They must cross what is called the blood-brain barrier, a membrane that extends across almost all of the brain and the spinal cord. It is an extremely effective barrier, and many substances cannot cross. Amino acids can enter the brain readily, but the bigger neurotransmitters derived from them cannot pass back into the bloodstream. Therefore, they cannot be directly measured by blood tests. Only by assessing their actions is it possible to deduce whether their supply is adequate.

The most important neurotransmitter in terms of feelings of well-being is serotonin. Adequate serotonin levels help us get to sleep at night and keep us calm during the day. Conversely, insufficient amounts of serotonin in the brain produce sleeplessness, anxiety, depression, and carbohydrate cravings.

Insulin has an additional action as well as its glucose-lowering and fat-building effects. It also lowers amino acids in the blood.

Of all the amino acids, only tryptophan remains relatively unaffected by insulin. Tryptophan can cross the blood-brain barrier without the usual competition from neighboring amino acids. It can then temporarily increase the production of the neurotransmitter serotonin, which produces a calming or comforting effect. Unfortunately, tryptophan's beneficial effects are only short-lived and lead to carbohydrate addiction because of the pleasure-seeking behavior that results from the consumption of simple carbohydrates. These cravings, common in obese patients, are the result of a deficiency of brain serotonin.

Here's an effective solution for you to discuss with your physician. The mild sleep aid trazodone can be very helpful for the insulin-resistant, carbohydrate-craving individual. Small doses of 25 to 200 milligrams of this safe medication have two distinct benefits. First, trazodone increases serotonin, which allows for better sleep at night. Second, the improved quality of sleep you'll enjoy elevates the body's production of serotonin.

The proper dose of trazodone is that which works for you, as indicated by control of carbohydrate cravings, improved sleep, and increased daytime energy. If your doctor agrees to provide you with a prescription for trazodone, you and your doctor can regulate the dosage to that which suits you best.

RELAXATION THROUGH DIURESIS

Beyond causing amino acid and neurotransmitter depletion, insulin resistance affects mood in other ways. As we have explained, high levels of insulin can lead to retention of salt and water. This can result in water intoxication, during which mental states deteriorate. In some cases patients can actually accumulate fluid in the brain, leading to swelling of the brain and subsequent mental abnormalities, including irritability, headaches, and the inability to think clearly. It is not safe to severely restrict salt because of the danger of postural hypotension (a drastic drop in blood pressure on standing that could lead to falling).

Our program of diet and exercise can do much to relieve the buildup of salt and water in the tissues. As insulin levels return to normal, the tendency to retain salt and water is diminished. To further enhance the removal of retained water, we recommend a technique known as diuresis of recumbency.

That might sound like a mouthful, but the concept is simple. Diuresis is the excretion of water from the tissues through the urine; *recumbency* means "a reclined position." The technique is a relaxing method of getting rid of built-up water by simply taking a rest. Here's how to do it.

Lie down on a bed or couch in an inclined rather than a completely prone position. Prop the upper part of your body up at a 45-degree angle with a few pillows. Relax in that position for about twenty minutes. You'll find that you arise refreshed and feeling the need to urinate. That's because the fluid has drained from your body's tissues and filled your bladder. The technique works by increasing the circulation to the kidneys, making them function more efficiently, with no depletion of potassium, which is an effect of most diuretics.

This is a useful technique that will help you get through those frustrating "plateau" periods when it seems that even though you are following the diet faithfully, the weight isn't coming off as fast as you'd like. Diuresis of recumbency helps to get the next few ounces of fluid out, and weight loss proceeds. And you'll enjoy the additional benefits of a brief period of relaxation while you are ridding the body of the excess fluid that can generate irritability and even depression.

RELAXATION THROUGH KETOSIS

While following this program, you'll find that ketosis produces a mild state of relaxation. No one understands exactly how this happens, but there's no question that almost every patient who enters and stays in ketosis experiences a calming effect. It's the desire to experience that kind of calm that leads people to take sedatives and tranquilizers. Unlike tranquilizers, though, ketosis calms without causing drowsiness or sluggishness.

It may well be that part of the "religious experience" of fasting may be due to the tranquilizing effects of the ketosis that would be generated by fasting.

People are as different on the inside as they are on the outside. Some seem to be born happy and are easily able to shrug off the blues. Others tend to be unhappy on a chronic basis and are often in a state of mild to moderate depression. Many authorities agree that the differences may come down to the fact that serotonin levels in the brain vary from person to person, just as other chemical substances in the body may vary.

Some chronically depressed individuals will certainly benefit from simply following this program of weight control, which, as an added benefit, increases serotonin levels and promotes calmness, serenity, and quality sleep. Others might need additional help but should not feel guilty about requiring medication to regulate a problem such as low serotonin levels any more than they would feel guilty about regulating a condition like insufficient thyroid hormone production.

Selective serotonin reuptake inhibitors (SSRIs) are a class of drugs that act to keep serotonin levels higher. The most frequently prescribed SSRI has been Prozac.

FOOD SENSITIVITIES

Some people find they can further elevate their moods by drinking coffee. The caffeine is, of course, a mild stimulant. In reasonable amounts caffeine can help you lose weight, working in the same way as amphetamines or other prescription drugs to depress appetite. By drinking coffee in small amounts, one can obtain the benefits of caffeine without the nerve-jangling adverse reactions of the notorious "diet pills." But the operative phrase here is "small amounts." Don't have more than two cups daily. And if even that amount starts to get you edgy, cut back to one cup.

Just as there are some people who react adversely to even the slightest bit of caffeine, certain individuals experience ill effects from other foods. Those physical reactions can definitely affect one's mood, especially if you don't know what's causing the problem.

One of the major offenders is milk. Many people cannot digest lactose, the sugar found in milk. Lactose-intolerant individuals do not produce enough of the enzyme lactase to break down the milk sugar into its two component simple sugars, glucose and galactose. The lactose remains in the digestive tract, begins to ferment, and leads to a variety of gastric symptoms. The symptoms may include flatulence, bloating, and diarrhea. The less lactase one produces, the more severe the symptoms can be. Since we hear so much about the "goodness" of milk, many of us never think to question the wisdom of its use for all people. The fact is that many people experience ill effects from drinking as little as one glass. This is especially true for blacks, Asians, and those of Mediterranean and Middle Eastern origin, but others develop the problem as well, particularly in adulthood.

During the weight loss phase of this program, milk is restricted. If you have regularly suffered gastric upset in the past, you may find that, for the first time in years, your symptoms go away. During the maintenance phase you may wish to start drinking milk again (skim milk, of course, because you certainly wouldn't want any extra fat and calories). If you find that gastric symptoms begin to recur, there are three solutions.

First, consider eliminating milk and perhaps other dairy foods from your diet. Calcium can be supplied by calcium carbonate tablets to reduce the potential development of osteoporosis. Second, try Lactaid, a brand of milk in which the lactose has been predigested by the addition of the enzyme lactase. Third, take lactase tablets, available in health food stores, after consuming dairy foods.

A similar kind of intolerance syndrome exists for some people who eat foods sweetened with sorbitol, a sugar substitute especially popular with diabetic patients who cannot tolerate sugar candy. Sorbitol-sweetened products include candies, gums, and other treats.

Intolerant individuals cannot break sorbitol down properly. As with lactose, it may remain in the digestive tract and begin to ferment. The result is a variety of symptoms including flatulence, bloating, and diarrhea. Symptoms may be mild to severe, and both children and adults may be afflicted. It's difficult to be in a good mood when one has such symptoms.

Some people must avoid sorbitol-sweetened products completely, but others may have a piece or two of such foods without an adverse reaction. During the first phase of this program, your carbohydrate intake will be greatly reduced, and such sweets will be eliminated. Later on you may choose to go back to sorbitol products. If so, let moderation be your rule.

RELIEF FROM PREMENSTRUAL SYNDROME

Patients afflicted with premenstrual syndrome (PMS) report mood swings, depression, irritability, anxiety, and a variety of other disturbed mental states. Authorities agree that diet plays a major role in the incidence and severity of PMS.

Patients with PMS often have an inordinate craving for carbohydrates. Since it is low in carbohydrates and high in protein, the diet you consume while following this program will be of enormous benefit if you suffer from PMS. Restricting carbohydrates helps to curb the craving for them, since, ironically, the more one eats, the more one wants. Abundant protein helps to improve neurotransmitter status, which is typically altered in those women complaining of PMS.

There is also a distinct tendency toward salt and water retention during PMS. Our diet will help eliminate puffiness, bloating, and irritability as well as the feeling that the brain is clouded, reported by many PMS victims.

Chapter 6

THE INSULIN CONTROL DIET

In the last nine years, after the initial weight loss of 64 pounds, my blood glucose, glycohemoglobin, insulin blood levels, and all other blood levels are normal or a little lower. My energy level is as good at age sixty-five as it was at forty-five. Though I am a Type 2 diabetic, I have been asymptomatic for eight and a half years. My weight has fluctuated less than 10 pounds. In short, I believe I have reversed my diabetes. Thank you very much.
—J.L., GRANADA HILLS, CALIFORNIA

You are about to learn the details of the Insulin Control Diet. It is a radical departure from the diets you've heard about, possibly tried from time to time, and with which you've routinely failed. When you have a lot to lose, the typical balanced diet, regardless of the number of calories provided, just will not take weight off effectively. You know that because you've tried time and time again, without any lasting success.

The weight loss program we advocate is not meant to be a permanent way of eating. It's a tested, effective method that, combined with the exercise advocated in Chapter 7, will help you reduce both pounds and inches safely and in a minimum amount of time.

Even before you begin to follow the program, read Chapter 10 on support. You'll learn how to motivate yourself, how to get over the rough spots, and in general how to gear up for success. As you learned in Chapter 4, most seriously overweight men and women have lost control of their bodies' endocrine balance. Excessive insulin produced by the pancreas has led to sodium and water retention, improper metabolism of sugars, and the inability to utilize the body's stored fatty acids. Within a short period of time, the Insulin Control Diet returns the body to normal endocrine control. Insulin production is greatly reduced, and the body uses the insulin that is produced more efficiently. Water and sodium are excreted rather than stored. And the body begins to break down its fat deposits, using that fat for energy.

The weight loss you experience during the first week or two will be dramatic because of the amount of water you'll be losing. Quite frankly, many diets do the same thing. Don't get too excited about it. But do get excited about the weight loss that invariably follows. Women can expect to lose up to 2 pounds each week. Men will lose up to 3 pounds weekly. Your rate of weight loss will depend on the amount of excess weight you're carrying, your age, the amount you exercise, and other individual differences.

The most significant aspect of your success with the Insulin Control Diet is that you will lose *fat*. That's not the case with far too many other diets, on which you also lose lean muscle tissue. That's so important that it deserves reiteration and emphasis here.

As we have explained, only muscle tissue has significant capability of burning calories, of using food for energy. Fat, on the other hand, is food—it cannot burn appreciable calories. Men typically can get away with eating more calories than women because they have a larger metabolic "engine" due to larger muscle mass. So you want to keep all the lean muscle you possibly can in order to burn calories most effectively now and in the future.

Lean muscle tissue also makes for a more attractive figure, for both men and women. Muscle gives us shape. As we replace fat tissue with lean tissue, we lose not only pounds but inches as well. You can measure your progress with both a scale and a tape measure.

Take your measurements today, before you start on the program. Measure your waist, hips, thighs, chest, and arms. You'll soon be seeing a dramatic difference. One of the most frequently cited thrills of those who have successfully lost weight with this program is seeing themselves in new clothes.

But there's an even more important reason for a diet that maintains lean muscle tissue. As we have said before, several well-known diets in the past have resulted in rapid loss of enormous amounts of weight. But much lean tissue was lost at the same time, and that muscle loss wasn't restricted to the arms or legs. Heart muscle was lost as well, and that led to cardiac arrhythmias (irregular heartbeats) that were sometimes fatal. When one starves to death, the actual cause of death is either heart failure or a lethal disturbance of heart rhythm (arrhythmia), owing to the loss of heart muscle tissue. The most notorious of such diets was the Last Chance Diet, which advocated a liquid protein diet. Sixty women actually died while following that program.

Medical authorities concerned with weight loss for greatly obese patients began developing protein-sparing diets to achieve rapid weight loss without significant loss of muscle. The Insulin Control Diet has brought these medically proven methods, employing low calorie diets, to the current state of the art. The most notable difference is that after just three days of adhering to the program, you will experience almost no hunger whatsoever. That's not idle speculation, but an observation based on years of clinical experience.

In the weeks to come you will consume as few as 1,000 calories for women and 1,500 for men daily. You'll lose water and fat during the first week or two, and lots and lots of fat in the weeks after that. Yet you won't be hungry. The reason is that while you're eating only approximately 1,000 to 1,500 calories daily, your body will be using about 2,000 to 2,500. The extra 1,000 to 1,500 calories will come directly from the fatty acids stored in your body in the form of adipose tissue. Your fatty acids will be released into the blood, where they will become your body's major source of fuel. And all the while you'll be consuming the right amounts of protein and fat for optimal nutrition as well as complete satisfaction.

For three days or less of following the Insulin Control Diet, the amount of insulin your body produces will drop dramatically, while the amount of glucagon will increase substantially. The body will produce ketones, which curb feelings of hunger. In the place of glucose or blood sugar, your body can also use those ketones as brain fuel, so that more precious protein can be spared.

One of the nice things about this aspect of the program is that you can observe directly how your body is adapting by measuring the degree of ketosis. (The use of KetoStix is described in Chapter 4.) Usually within three days of following the program the KetoStix will turn a shade ranging from pink to purple, indicating that you've entered a state of mild ketosis. On the Insulin Control Diet, the ketosis remains mild, never developing to a state severe enough to pose potential damage.

As stated earlier, the Number One Poison for overweight people is sugar. Even the slightest amount of simple sugars in the diet causes an increased flow of insulin. Until the body's endocrine balance becomes restored, both simple sugars such as table sugar and complex carbohydrates such as pasta, cereals, and fruits will result in the same insidious cycle of insulin release, insulin resistance, sodium and fluid retention, fat storage, weight gain, and depression. For a brief time, it is necessary to restrict severely the amount of *all* carbohydrates entering the body. The body must be given a rest so that eventually it can discriminate between nutritious carbohydrates and bloating sugars.

While the diet we're proposing may at first appear radical, ask yourself if you wouldn't be able to deal with some temporary deprivation if you were given the virtual guarantees that (1) you will be able to lose fat more effectively than ever before, (2) you will do so without hunger, and (3) you will be able to maintain that weight loss for the rest of your life. Those are the guarantees the Insulin Control Diet has to offer.

The diet is divided into three phases: weight loss, stabilization, and maintenance. How long you will be in the first phase depends on how much weight you have to lose. If you have more than 50 pounds to lose, you may shed between 8 and 10 pounds of combined water and fat during the first two weeks. Thereafter, you may lose up to 2 pounds a week if you're a woman and up to 3 pounds a week if you're a man, until you've reached your goal. You can see that the Insulin Control Diet gets you to your ideal weight within a reasonable period of time. You'll then enter the stabilization phase, in which you'll learn to keep your weight constant, neither gaining nor losing, while eating a variety of foods. And finally, you'll learn the techniques of weight maintenance, assuring a lifetime of optimum weight and health.

The diet itself is remarkably simple. You won't have to count calories, read complex charts, or rely on specific foods. The entire regimen has been scientifically designed to provide good nutrition, with all the nutrients your body needs and in a way that will put you on the track to wise food choices for the rest of your life.

For the duration of your weight loss period, we ask that you limit your total carbohydrate intake to 20 to 30 grams. This means that, for a limited period of time, you will have to eliminate a great number of the foods you've become accustomed to and that, under other circumstances, are excellent, nutritious foods.

On the Insulin Control Diet, what you do not eat is far more important than what you do eat. In other words, more than 30 grams of carbohydrate in any form will trigger your overproduction of insulin and return you to the weight gain cycle you know so well. Isn't it worth it to do without breads and pastas and to cut down on fruits and starchy vegetables for a while, knowing that this diet will absolutely and positively eliminate your weight problem?

We recommend you divide your allocated calories into three meals and two snacks. This establishes a healthful eating pattern. Eating all your food in two meals creates insulin and blood sugar spikes, which prevents weight loss. Also, it is important to spread out your carbohydrates during the day. We recommend not exceeding 8 grams carbohydrates per meal and 4 grams carbohydrates per snack, in order to stay in ketosis. Try to eat breakfast, even if you haven't been doing so in the past. A protein shake, used as a meal replacement for breakfast, is a convenient and effective weight loss aid as well. Choose between Atkins Advantage and Worldwide Pure Protein shakes.

We'd like you to get into the healthful habit of drinking lots of fluids throughout the day. Fluids will help satisfy your need for oral satisfaction in place of some of the snacking you've been doing in the past. At the same time they flush out wastes into your urine. Water is still the best fluid to consume, but you may also wish to include diet sodas, iced tea, herbal teas, decaffeinated coffee, and club soda or mineral waters, for a total of at least eight 8-ounce glasses daily. While it's true that most diet sodas contain no carbohydrates and no calories, they may remind you of other sweets. As much as possible, start switching from artificially sweetened sodas to club soda and seltzers and mineral water, perhaps flavored with a twist of lemon or orange.

For a particularly elegant drink, try serving mineral or sparkling water over ice in a large wine goblet. And here's a special bartender's trick: Twist an orange peel over a lighted match to release a drop or two of the orange oil into the drink. The oil will flame and sizzle momentarily, releasing a lovely burnt orange flavor. Since no alcohol is permitted during your weight loss period, this makes a nice substitute for a social cocktail. Until you are well established in maintenance, with weight loss secure, avoid alcohol. It interferes with achieving endocrine balance, and its 7 calories per gram are empty calories. (See the table in the Appendix for the caloric content of various alcoholic beverages.) Today there's a definite trend away from the heavy use of alcohol. Get on the bandwagon.

You will gradually come to enjoy drinking healthful amounts of water. Journalists often say that their typewriters "run" on a perpetual flow of coffee. What they're saying is that they're in the habit of sipping as they sit at their computers. While the caffeine in coffee can jangle the nerves and perhaps contribute to health problems, the coffee mug can be filled with other fluids to satisfy the same pleasant sipping habit.

We've included snacks in the program, but since sugar is the Number One Poison, you want to eliminate refined sugars entirely. To satisfy a sweet tooth on occasion, we suggest sugar-free gelatin. Keep a good supply on hand, and keep some prepared in your refrigerator. For variety, try preparing different flavors and colors and adding fruits or salad greens as your meal plan allows. (Some recipe suggestions are given in Chapter 11.) Many patients say that gelatin desserts are lifesavers, keeping them going during the first weeks of the Insulin Control Diet. Just knowing such a dessert is in the refrigerator gives comfort. And even after the weight loss period, patients continue to enjoy this "insulin right" snack.

Lettuce, celery, and leafy greens, such as spinach and cabbage, can also be eaten in large amounts on the program. Limit yourself to one full head of lettuce or its equivalent each day. The greens add few carbohydrates to your total dietary plan, and they provide lots of fiber and satisfaction. Leafy greens are also definitely insulin right foods.

Since regular breads are not permitted during the weight loss period of the Insulin Control Diet, lettuce comes to the rescue. When you crave a sandwich, wrap some meat, a bit of onion, and a dash of pepper sauce in two large leaves of romaine lettuce instead of using bread. Sauces and condiments that add zing to your sandwich without adding too many carbohydrates include mustard, horseradish, and some salad dressings. (The composition of some salad dressings is given in the table in the Appendix.) Low carb bread (one slice) is permitted, including brands such as Oroweat Light, Sara Lee Delightful, and Weight Watchers.

Carbohydrate content is the most important consideration in determining insulin right and insulin wrong foods.

Be advised that regardless of total calories consumed, carbohydrate intake for the day should fall within 25 to 30 grams, having no more than 8 to 10 grams carbohydrates at any one meal and no more than 5 grams of carbohydrates per snack.

During the weight loss period you'll be eating large quantities of protein-rich foods, including meats, fish and other seafood, and poultry. First, these foods provide nourishment without carbohydrates. Second, and most important, they supply a defense against protein loss from muscle tissue normally seen in rapid weight loss, especially during fasting.

> **D**uring weight loss you'll be eating more protein foods than you would normally consider part of a balanced diet.

THE FREE FOOD LIST

Although these foods contain very low amounts of carbohydrates, if any at all, the term "free" must be considered within reason.

Vegetables

Cabbage (all varieties), raw	Dill pickles, 2–4
Spinach, raw	Endive
Zucchini, raw	Green onion
Mushrooms, raw	Hot peppers
Lettuce (all varieties)	Radishes
Celery	Watercress
Cucumber	

Drinks

Chicken broth	Club soda
Tea, decaf or regular	Diet green tea
Coffee, decaf preferable	Carb-free flavored water

Sweets

Reddi-wip whipped cream
Sugar-free gelatin (Please limit
  consumption; no more than
  a few a week; contains
  aspartame.)

Stevia
Splenda

Condiments and Seasonings

Herbs (basil, mint, oregano,
  etc.)
Horseradish
Mustard
Soy sauce
Vinegar

Salad dressing (1–2 grams
  carbohydrates)
Spices (celery seeds, curry,
  cinnamon)
Extracts (vanilla, etc.)

Sugar-Free Gum

3 pieces a day (no more than 1
  gram carbohydrates per piece)

ADDITIONAL RECOMMENDATIONS

We strongly recommend eating only lean meats and trimming all visible fat from meat servings. Moreover, we believe that during the first few weeks of your weight loss period you will be better off with little red meat (no more than once a week), relying instead on fish and poultry. Use cooking methods that call for little added oil. Enjoy your foods baked, broiled, steamed, poached, and boiled rather than fried or sautéed. When you want to use the frying pan, use a nonstick pan and a light application of vegetable oil spray, or use a tablespoon or two of bouillon to keep food from sticking.

Are you a dessert addict? As we mentioned, sugar-free gelatin can be satisfying and has helped keep many a dieter faithful to the program. You may also save your fruit serving for dessert. When enjoying a gelatin dessert or fruit, you might want to make it more festive with a dab of Reddi-wip. Little touches such as these can make the weight loss experience so much more pleasant. If you whiten your coffee with cream or nondairy creamer, try a dab of either one of these products there as well. You'll have all the satisfaction without fat and carbohydrates.

Since during the period of weight loss your body will be eliminating great amounts of both water and sodium, you will want to add enough sodium to your diet to prevent a potential sodium shortage. Try using a total of 1 teaspoonful of salt each day in cooking or as seasoning.

All individuals participating in the weight loss program need to add 1 teaspoon of salt (= 200 milligrams sodium) throughout the day, including individuals who are taking blood pressure medications. The program lowers your insulin levels, causing a natural diuretic effect (fluid loss). If you do not consume extra salt, you may be at risk of very low blood pressure, causing dizziness or light-headedness, as well as at risk of dehydration and electrolyte imbalances. In addition to 1 teaspoon of salt throughout the day, you must drink eight to ten 8-ounce cups of water a day to prevent dehydration.

Remember, you need 2,000 milligrams sodium per day.

Suggestions for High Salt Food Choices

6 olives
2 slices cold cuts turkey (= 400 milligrams sodium)
½ cup cottage cheese (= 400 milligrams sodium)
2 dill pickles with no sugar added
Soy sauce
1 cup chicken bouillon broth (= 800–1,000 milligrams sodium)
Salt from the shaker (¼ teaspoon = 500 milligrams sodium)

Since the Insulin Control Diet greatly limits the total amount of food you consume daily, albeit without any hunger, it's more difficult to obtain all the vitamins, minerals, and trace nutrients your body requires, so we recommend you take a daily multiple vitamin and mineral supplement. Since foods rich in potassium have been eliminated during the weight loss period, potassium supplements may be appropriate. This is particularly true for dieters with high blood pressure currently taking diuretic drugs. A very convenient way to add potassium to the diet is to use one of the salt substitutes, which replace sodium with potassium. Simply sprinkle some of the salt substitute on your food daily. However, if you are currently taking diuretic drugs due to high blood pressure, by all means, consult your physician about using salt substitutes.

For women, the total calorie content of the following meal plan each day is about 1,000 calories. For men, the total is about 1,100–1,500 calories. Men require slightly more protein and extra calories because their muscle mass and hence their metabolic engines are larger than women's. Remember that in addition to the calories provided by the food you eat, you'll be consuming your own stored supplies of fatty acids to meet your energy requirements. That will add about an extra 1,000–1,800 calories daily. You'll be completely satisfied and never hungry, especially after ketone production has begun. That's how your fat can help you become thin!

We have listed a full two weeks of meal plans, including three meals and two snacks for each day. The items marked with an asterisk are included in the recipe section in Chapter 11. When you've gone through the fifteen meal plans, you may simply repeat them through the weight loss phase, or you may prefer to interchange menu items. There are enough food suggestions to keep you satisfied for months.

Each day, measure your progress by checking the color change on your KetoStix. Each week, measure your improvement in inches and in pounds on the bathroom scale. Nothing breeds success like success; your 2-, 3-, or 4-pound weekly loss will encourage you to continue. During the weight loss phase of this program, we recommend that you weigh yourself only weekly. That may come as a surprise, but we have good reason for this advice. We can confidently predict up to 2 pounds of weight loss weekly for women and up to 3 pounds for men. Individual loss will, of course, vary. But the loss on a daily basis will vary considerably for each person. One day you might see significant loss, while another day produces no progress whatsoever. That can be frustrating. Avoid the temptation of daily weighing and stick to the weekly schedule.

Before you begin the program, make a contract with yourself that you will continue it all the way to the end. Don't settle for a 20-pound loss when a 35-pound loss is what you want and need. As we have said, those who quit midway through the program have no chance of reaching their ideal weights, and they have the least chance of keeping off whatever weight they do lose. Those who stay with the program can reach their goals and maintain their ideal weights.

Start planning now. Decide what you'll have for breakfast tomorrow morning, for lunch, for dinner, and for the next several meals; then make your shopping list. Pick up a supply of KetoStix and your calcium and vitamin and mineral supplements on your way to the supermarket. For help, review the weight loss checklist.

Weight Loss Phase: A Checklist

- Total daily calories: 1,000 for women; 1,100–1,500 for men
- Total daily carbohydrate: 20–30 grams (maximum 40 grams) of complex carbohydrates; no simple sugars
- Total daily protein: 55–75 grams from 7–10 ounces of fish, poultry (skinless), or lean meat (fat trimmed) plus 1 egg or 2 ounces of low-fat cottage cheese
- ½ cup raw free veggies each day
- ½ cup of vegetable each day from the vegetable list (not the starchy vegetables on the starch and bread list)
- 1 slice of light whole wheat low carbohydrate bread each day
- A protein shake with no more than 5 total carbohydrates each day
- 1 low carbohydrate yogurt: Dannon Lite & Fit Carb & Sugar Control or Ralphs Carb Master
- 15–20 almonds; small servings of avocados, as they have lots of calories
- Calcium supplement (1,000 milligrams) with vitamin D
- Multiple vitamin and mineral pill (100 percent RDA)
- 1 teaspoon of salt in cooking or as seasoning
- Vitamin B_{12} (1,000 micrograms sublingual)
- Cook without fat or use vegetable oil spray.
- Drink eight to ten 8-ounce glasses of fluid, preferably water, each day.
- Follow the two-week menu plan (pages 71–85), varying items.
- Monitor ketosis with KetoStix before and after bedtime.
- Weigh on scale weekly.

As you look over the meal plans, imagine that you're glancing at the menu of an expensive, world-famous health spa. The menus and the recipes in Chapter 11 are in fact similar to the foods served at those exclusive enclaves. You're getting the very best that money can buy. And you deserve it!

Remember, our goal is to give your body a temporary break from most carbohydrates. The following list of Foods to Avoid and Your Carbohydrate Counter for Weight Loss will help you achieve this goal.

FOODS TO AVOID

Avoid the following: Fruit (except ½ cup berries), juice, all milk (except Almond Breeze unsweetened), cereal, oatmeal, protein bars, nuts (except 15–20 almonds or cashews as a snack per day), corn, peas, potatoes, beets, carrots, beans, rice, pasta, breads (except low carb), pastries, flour, sugar, honey, dried fruit, soup (bouillon is OK).

Your Carbohydrate Counter for Weight Loss

½ cup berries = 8 grams carbohydrates
½ cup vegetables = 5 grams carbohydrates (exception: free vegetables)
1 slice low carbohydrate bread = 8–9 grams carbohydrates
1 protein shake = 5 grams carbohydrates
Low carb yogurt = 3–4 grams carbohydrates
Dannon Lite & Fit Carb & Sugar Control yogurt = 3 grams carbohydrates (Gelson's)
Ralphs Carbmaster yogurt = 4 grams carbohydrates
FAGE 0% or 2%Greek yogurt = 7–8 grams carbohydrates
½ cup low fat cottage cheese = 4 grams
  • Low Fat Organic Horizon Cottage Cheese (Gelson's or Whole Foods)
  • Lucerne Low Fat Cottage Cheese (Vons)
  • Low Fat Organic Cottage Cheese (Trader Joe's)
  • Alta Dena Cottage Cheese (Gelson's)

Do not count carbohydrate grams from protein foods like eggs, cheese, chicken, fish, turkey, and seafood. Just be observant of the portion sizes specified in your menu. Also, stay away from beef, pork, lamb, whole fat cheese, nuts, and avocados, and use only reduced calorie salad dressing. Furthermore, do not combine any two low carbohydrate food items; rather, combine one low carbohydrate food with one lean protein item.

MEAL PLAN—DAY ONE

Thought for the day: The journey of a thousand miles begins with a single step.

Breakfast

Decaffeinated coffee or herbal tea
1–2 poached eggs or 1 cup egg substitute
1 cup chicken or beef bouillon broth
½–¾ cup low fat cottage cheese

Snack

1 low fat string cheese and ½ cup berries

Lunch

Iced tea or mineral water with lemon twist
Chicken Breast Mexicali* (4 ounces for women, 5 ounces for men)
Salad with Low-Cal Vinaigrette dressing*
Checkerboard Gelatin*

Snack

3 stalks celery and reduced fat garden vegetable cream cheese

Dinner

Indian Fish Curry* (5 ounces for women, 6 ounces for men)
¾ cup Asparagus Chinese Style*
2–3 cups salad with Dill Vinaigrette dressing*
1 cup chicken or beef broth
Gelatin with Reddi-wip whipped cream

*See recipe section.

Additional fluids as desired to complete minimum of eight 8-ounce
servings daily

MEAL PLAN—DAY TWO

Thought for the day: Plan a special treat—a bubble bath perhaps—
for taking such good care of yourself.

Breakfast

Decaffeinated coffee or herbal tea
1–2 soft cooked eggs or ½ cup egg substitute
2 slices turkey bacon
1 slice low carbohydrate bread (e.g., Sara Lee Delightful or Oroweat
Light = 9 grams carbohydrates)

Snack

2 slices turkey cold cuts
1–2 pickles
Chicken or beef broth

Lunch

Iced coffee or diet soda
Salmon Salad Sandwich* (4 ounces for women, 5 ounces for men)
Salad with Low-Cal Vinaigrette dressing*
Gelatin with Reddi-wip whipped cream

Snack

15–20 flavored nuts (e.g., Blue Diamond Salt & Vinegar or Wasabi
& Soy Sauce)

Dinner

Decaffeinated coffee or tea
Chinese Fish Steak* (5 ounces for women, 6 ounces for men)
Beans with Basil*
Salad with Parsley Vinaigrette dressing*

1–2 pieces of Lindt Excellence 85% Cocoa Chocolate, 3 pieces 70% Green & Black's chocolate, or 1–2 wedges 70% Coca dark chocolate

Additional fluids as desired to complete minimum of eight 8-ounce servings daily

MEAL PLAN—DAY THREE

Thought for the day: Call a friend to tell her or him how excited you are that you found the answer to your diet problems.

Breakfast

Decaffeinated coffee or tea

2-egg or egg substitute omelet with ¾ cup bell pepper and mushrooms

1 slice Swiss cheese melted over omelet

Snack

2 wedges Laughing Cow Light Cheese

½–¾ cup baby tomatoes

1–2 small cucumbers

Lunch

Mineral water with a lemon twist or iced tea

Chicken Cobb Salad* (4 ounces chicken for women, 5 ounces chicken for men)

1–2 pieces of Lindt Excellence 85% Cocoa Chocolate, 3 pieces 70% Green & Black's chocolate, or 1–2 wedges 70% Coca dark chocolate

Snack

Ralphs Carb Master yogurt or ½ cup cottage cheese

Dinner

Decaffeinated coffee or tea

Florentine Chicken* (5 ounces for women, 6 ounces for men)

Salad with Curry Vinaigrette dressing*
1 cup chicken bouillon broth
Additional fluids as desired to complete minimum of eight 8-ounce
 servings daily

MEAL PLAN—DAY FOUR

Thought for the day: As you enter ketosis, you no longer feel hungry. Your mind is free to think about so many things other than food!

Breakfast

Decaffeinated coffee or herbal tea
Chilled Atkins shake or low carb Slim-Fast shake
1 hard cooked egg or ½ cup egg substitute

Snack

½ cup raspberries and 2 tablespoons Reddi-wip whipped cream

Lunch

Green salad with a scoop of tuna (light mayonnaise)
½ cup baby tomatoes
Dill pickle
½ cup bamboo shoots

Snack

FAGE 0% or 2% Greek yogurt or Ralphs Carb Master yogurt

Dinner

Decaffeinated coffee or tea
Chinese Chicken Stir-Fry* (5 ounces chicken for women, 6 ounces
 chicken for men)
Salad with Curry Vinaigrette dressing*
1 cup chicken bouillon broth
Gelatin "Cookies"*

Additional fluids as desired to complete minimum of eight 8-ounce
servings daily

MEAL PLAN—DAY FIVE

Thought for the day: Look in the mirror and smile at the person you
see; give yourself all the love and acceptance you can.

Breakfast

Decaffeinated coffee or herbal tea
2 low fat turkey sausages
¾ cup low fat cottage cheese
1 cup chicken or beef bouillon broth

Snack

½ cup raspberries
Low fat string cheese

Lunch

Mineral water with a squeeze of lime
Sautéed Chicken Breast* (4 ounces for women, 5 ounces for men)
Checkerboard Gelatin*

Snack

EAS AdvantEdge protein shake or AchievONE protein shake

Dinner

Decaffeinated coffee or tea
Salmon in Court Bouillon* (5 ounces for women, 6 ounces for
men)
½ cup cut up bell pepper
Salad with Mexican Vinaigrette dressing*
1 cup chicken bouillon broth
Additional fluids as desired to complete minimum of eight 8-ounce
servings daily

MEAL PLAN—DAY SIX

Thought for the day: Recall the fond memories of your life that are not about food; remember what made these times happy.

Breakfast

Decaffeinated coffee or herbal tea
1–2 sunnyside-up eggs or ¼–½ cup egg substitute
½ cup sautéed mushrooms and ½ cup sautéed bell pepper or onion
1 cup chicken bouillon broth
1–2 small cucumbers

Snack

½ protein shake (e.g., low carb Slim-Fast)
1 piece low carbohydrate chocolate

Lunch

Diet soda
Poultry Burger* (4 ounces for women, 5 ounces for men)
Small salad with Low-Cal Vinaigrette dressing*

Snack

½ protein shake
1 piece low carbohydrate chocolate

Dinner

Decaffeinated coffee or herbal tea
New Orleans Creole Fillet* (5 ounces for women, 6 ounces for men)
¾ cup cabbage
Dinner salad with Dill Vinaigrette dressing*
1 cup chicken bouillon broth
Checkerboard Gelatin*
Additional fluids as desired to complete minimum of eight 8-ounce
  servings daily

MEAL PLAN—DAY SEVEN

Thought for the day: Weight control is worth a *fortune* in good health and happiness. You're getting *rich*!

Breakfast

Chilled protein shake (Atkins or low carb Slim-Fast!)
½ cup egg white salad

Snack

1 low fat string cheese
½ cup berries

Lunch

Mineral water with lemon twist
Cold shrimp with Low-Cal Vinaigrette dressing* (4 ounces shrimp for women, 5 ounces shrimp for men)
1 cup chopped tomato cucumber salad with Parsley Vinaigrette dressing*

Snack

½ cup cottage cheese mixed with Splenda (or Stevia) and cinnamon

Dinner

Decaffeinated coffee or tea
Poultry Meatloaf* (5 ounces for women, 6 ounces for men)
½ cup broccoli florets, steamed or boiled
Small salad with Parsley Vinaigrette dressing*
1 cup beef bouillon broth
Gelatin Salad*
Additional fluids as desired to complete minimum of eight 8-ounce servings daily

MEAL PLAN—DAY EIGHT

Thought for the day: Many, many people are on diets for one reason or another; you're in good company.

Breakfast

Decaffeinated coffee or tea
1–2 deviled eggs or ½ cup egg substitute
¾ cup salsa
1 cup chicken bouillon broth

Snack

¾ cup strawberries

Lunch

Diet soda
Poultry Meatloaf* (leftover from yesterday's dinner: 4 ounces for
    women, 5 ounces for men)
Gelatin Salad* (leftover from yesterday's dinner)

Snack

3 stalks of celery and reduced fat garden vegetable cream cheese

Dinner

Decaffeinated coffee or tea
Chicken à l'Orange* (5 ounces for women, 6 ounces for men)
Salad with Dill Vinaigrette dressing*
1 cup beef bouillon broth
Gelatin and Reddi-wip whipped cream
Additional fluids as desired to complete minimum of eight 8-ounce
    servings daily

MEAL PLAN—DAY NINE

Thought for the day: You're well into the second week of the program. Congratulations! It only gets easier.

Breakfast

Decaffeinated coffee or tea
1–2 poached eggs or ¼–½ cup egg substitute
1 cup beef bouillon broth
Ralphs Carb Master yogurt

Snack

Emerald 100-calorie pack Cocoa Roast Almonds (4 grams
    carbohydrate)

Lunch

Mineral water with orange twist
Italian Poultry Burger* (4 ounces for women, 5 ounces for men)
Gelatin "Cookies"*

Snack

½–¾ cup baby tomatoes

Dinner

Decaffeinated coffee or tea
This 'n' That Seafood Soup* (5 ounces for women, 6 ounces for men)
½ artichoke
Salad with Low-Cal Vinaigrette dressing*
1 cup beef bouillon broth
Additional fluids as desired to complete minimum of eight 8-ounce
    servings daily

MEAL PLAN—DAY TEN

Thought for the day: Make a resolution to continue to succeed, no
matter what the occasion. No piece of cake or treat is worth blowing
it now.

Breakfast

Decaffeinated coffee or tea
1 egg or ¼ cup egg substitute scrambled with cubed, low fat turkey
    sausage and chives

1 slice low carbohydrate bread (e.g., Sara Lee Delightful or Oroweat Light)

Spread with Walden Farms 0 gram carbohydrate jam, or any sugar-free jam

Snack

1–2 turkey cold cut rollups with Swiss cheese
Sugar-free green tea

Lunch

Iced tea sweetened with Splenda or Stevia
Salmon Salad Sandwich* (4 ounces for women, 5 ounces for men)
Checkerboard Gelatin*

Snack

15–20 flavored nuts (e.g., Blue Diamond Salt & Vinegar or Wasabi & Soy Sauce)

Dinner

Decaffeinated coffee or tea
Turkey Cutlet* (5 ounces for women, 6 ounces for men)
¾ cup cabbage
Salad with Dill Vinaigrette dressing*
1 cup chicken bouillon broth
Gelatin with Reddi-wip whipped cream
Additional fluids as desired to complete minimum of eight 8-ounce servings daily

MEAL PLAN—DAY ELEVEN

Thought for the day: Think about the diet as a hobby—be creative about your salads and gelatin desserts.

Breakfast

Decaffeinated coffee or tea
1–2 soft boiled eggs or ¼–½ cup egg substitute

2 pieces turkey bacon or turkey sausage
½ cup bell pepper

Snack

½ cup blueberries
1 low fat string cheese

Lunch

Mineral water with a squeeze of lime
Turkey Cutlet* (leftover from yesterday's dinner: 4 ounces for
    women, 5 ounces for men)
Gelatin Salad*

Snack

3 stalks celery and reduced fat garden vegetable cream cheese
Sugar-free green tea (e.g., Hansen's green tea)

Dinner

Decaffeinated coffee or tea
Salmon Chowder* (5 ounces for women, 6 ounces for men)
Salad with Parsley Vinaigrette dressing*
1 cup chicken bouillon broth
Gelatin Salad*
Additional fluids as desired to complete minimum of eight 8-ounce
    servings daily

MEAL PLAN—DAY TWELVE

Thought for the day: Remember the days when you were more slender and the things you used to enjoy. Soon you'll enjoy them again.

Breakfast

Decaffeinated coffee or tea
Chicken salad with celery, chives, and light mayonnaise

½ cup baby tomatoes
1 cup chicken bouillon broth

Snack

3–4 halves deviled eggs
1–2 dill pickles

Lunch

Diet soda or iced tea
Tuna salad sandwich (4 ounces for women, 5 ounces for men)
3 stalks celery
Gelatin "Cookies"*

Snack

15–20 Blue Diamond Almonds, Smoke Flavored

Dinner

Decaffeinated coffee or tea
Oriental Ginger Fish* (5 ounces for women, 6 ounces for men)
¾ cup Asparagus Chinese Style*
Salad with Low-Cal Vinaigrette dressing*
1 cup beef bouillon broth
Additional fluids as desired to complete minimum of eight 8-ounce
    servings daily

MEAL PLAN—DAY THIRTEEN

Thought for the day: Sometimes your best friend can be your worst
enemy by talking you into a treat "just this once." Stand by your
plan.

Breakfast

Decaffeinated coffee or tea
1–2 basted eggs or ¼–½ cup egg substitute
FAGE 0% Greek yogurt, plain
1 cup beef bouillon broth

Snack

½ cup raspberries
1 low fat string cheese

Lunch

Mineral water with lemon twist
Cold crab meat (snow crab, Dungeness crab, etc.; 4 ounces for
    women, 5 ounces for men)
Gelatin Salad*

Snack

1–2 turkey cold cut rollups with Swiss cheese

Dinner

Decaffeinated coffee or tea
Oven "Fried" Scallops* (5 ounces for women, 6 ounces for men)
Beans with Basil*
Salad with Curry Vinaigrette dressing*
1 cup chicken bouillon
Gelatin with Reddi-wip whipped cream
Additional fluids as desired to complete minimum of eight 8-ounce
    servings daily

MEAL PLAN—DAY FOURTEEN

Thought for the day: You've made it through two whole weeks, and
your weight loss shows it. Congratulations!

Breakfast

Decaffeinated coffee or tea
1–2 scrambled eggs or ½ cup egg substitute
1–2 turkey sausages
1 cup chicken bouillon broth
½ cup low fat cottage cheese mixed with Splenda or Stevia and
    cinnamon

Snack

2 tablespoons whipped cream cheese
½ cup raspberries

Lunch

Diet soda
Oriental Poultry Burger* (4 ounces for women, 5 ounces for men)
Romaine lettuce
Gelatin with chocolate Reddi-wip whipped cream

Snack

Ralphs Carb Master yogurt or ½ cup low fat cottage cheese

Dinner

Decaffeinated coffee or tea
Beef en Brochette* (5 ounces for women, 6 ounces for men)
Salad with Dill Vinaigrette dressing*
1 cup beef bouillon broth
Checkerboard Gelatin*
Additional fluids as desired to complete minimum of eight 8-ounce
    servings daily

MEAL PLAN—DAY FIFTEEN AND BEYOND

Thought for the day: Keep a positive attitude that the rest of your diet program will go smoothly. Consult the suggestions in Chapter 10 on support regularly.

Breakfast

Decaffeinated coffee or tea
Protein shake
1 cup beef or chicken bouillon broth

Snack

½ cup egg white salad
½ cup berries

Lunch

Diet green tea
1 protein entrée of your choice (4 ounces for women, 5 ounces for men)
Green salad with vinaigrette dressing of your choice

Snack

1 low fat string cheese
1–2 pieces low carbohydrate chocolate

Dinner

Decaffeinated coffee or tea
1 protein entrée of your choice (fish and poultry, with red meat once a week; 5 ounces for women, 6 ounces for men)
Salad with vinaigrette dressing of your choice
1 cup beef or chicken bouillon broth
Gelatin dessert
Additional fluids as desired to complete minimum of eight 8-ounce servings daily

COMMONLY ASKED QUESTIONS

Q: *Are all kinds of meats and poultry OK on this diet?*
A: Raw, unprocessed meats of all kinds are totally free of carbohydrates. However, be sure to read the Nutrition Facts label on all processed meats such as sausages and luncheon meats.
Q: *Is it OK to shoot for zero carbohydrates during the first few days to simplify things?*
A: It's actually not all that easy to achieve a true "zero-carb" diet. You'll find a few grams here and a few grams there, and they do add up. But, yes, to make things easier during the first few days as you get into ketosis it's fine to limit carbohydrates entirely. As you become more familiar with the diet, begin to follow the daily meal plans we've provided.
Q: *I began the diet but it took five days to see a reading on the KetoStix indicating I'd entered ketosis. Is that normal?*

A: The time to enter ketosis varies from person to person. It does not depend on gender, age, fitness, or amount of overweight. The range of time can be anywhere from two days to even six days.

Q: *Will I be hungry during the time it takes to reach ketosis?*

A: Some people find that they're not hungry even before the Keto-Stix begins to show one has entered ketosis.

Q: *What does it take to get out of ketosis?*

A: Again, depending on the individual it can take as little as one carbohydrate-rich meal (more than 8 grams of carbohydrates) to throw one out of ketosis. Other people can slip a bit and remain in ketosis.

Q: *Once I'm out of ketosis, say after a weekend splurge, how long will it take to get back?*

A: Unfortunately, it sometimes takes longer to get back into ketosis than it did originally. That's a good reason to try one's best to be compliant with the diet throughout the weight loss period.

Q: *Since I'm sleeping poorly, should I start taking a higher dose of trazodone?*

A: No. Begin with just half a tablet. If, after a week, you find that isn't enough, increase the dosage under your doctor's direction to a full tablet. Make increases in half-tablet increments under your doctor's direction.

Q: *Will I need more trazodone as time goes on?*

A: Happily, one does not form a tolerance to trazodone as one might to other agents. If anything, you may find you'll need smaller amounts as time goes on.

Q: *Do you have e-mail so your readers can reach you directly?*

A: Our e-mail is ezrincenter@aol.com. Do feel free to write to us let us know how you are doing.

Q: *Will my menstrual period affect my level of ketosis?*

A: Stress hormones are increased during one's period. Substances such as cortisol, adrenaline, growth hormone, and glucagon can elevate blood sugar unless more insulin is secreted. Insulin will tend to diminish ketosis by reducing liberation of fatty acids.

Q: *My teenaged daughter is about 20 pounds overweight. Is this dietary program recommended for teens or only adults?*

A: We have successfully treated teens in our center. However, this program should be carefully monitored, and I would not recommend your daughter do it on her own.

Q: *Can I save carbohydrates through the day in order to have them all at one meal?*

A: It's the total number of grams of carbohydrates per meal that matters most. One should not exceed 8 grams of carbohydrates at any one meal in order to remain in ketosis. Individual thresholds for maximum carbohydrates per meal vary, and some people may afford to go up to about 12 grams of carbohydrates per meal. Let ketosis be your "litmus test."

Q: *How much water and how much fat will be in the total weight loss, especially at the beginning?*

A: Of the first 6 pounds, let's say, 3 to 4 pounds will be water. As time goes on, the ratio will improve until the majority of the weight loss is fat rather than water.

Q: *How important is the daily log?*

A: We find that those who really keep a scrupulous log or diary do much better than those who don't. Writing down your food and beverage intake, exercise, trazodone dosage, sleep patterns, and state of ketosis provides tremendous motivation.

Q: *Can I switch dinner and lunch?*

A: Switching lunch and dinner is highly encouraged in our program. This switch produces faster weight loss and much better blood sugar control in the morning. But why is this? One of the reasons is that the typical protein size (ounces) for dinner is larger than at lunch, which results in consuming more calories at dinner. Digesting more calories at night tends to put ketosis on "pause," which slows weight loss. In addition, heavier proteins, such as beef, lamb, and pork, may take as long as seven hours to digest. We teach our patients to choose these proteins only once or twice a week and preferably for lunch. Furthermore, carbohydrates will be absorbed from cooked vegetables at dinner. To summarize, choose chicken or fish, and occasionally beef or pork, for lunch, along with ¾ cup cooked vegetables. Choose salad and a few ounces of lean protein for dinner. Preferable dinner proteins are the light ones that take only two to three hours to digest, such as 2–3 ounces tuna salad, egg white salad, or chicken breast; 3 ounces tofu; or ¾ cup cottage cheese. A protein shake can even be used once in a while as a dinner replacement. However, do not replace more than one meal per day with a protein shake.

Q: *Is it OK to skip breakfast?*
A: Research shows that skipping breakfast slows down your metabolism. For convenience, have a protein shake.
Q: *Can I have a snack during the day?*
A: You should have two snacks per day on this program. You can also have celery, cucumbers, and other "free" vegetables at any time. When snacking between meals, select low carbohydrate foods such as cut-up celery, cucumbers, zucchini, and radishes dipped into a blend of low fat cottage cheese and herbs or low calorie salad dressing. For more suggestions, refer to the snack list at the end of this chapter. Sip some broth with some greens tossed in. Enjoy fat-free lunch meat slices, or low fat cheese slices.
Q: *Do I need to have the salt?*
A: Salt is certainly important on this diet. When you are on a low carbohydrate diet, insulin, which retains salt and water, is not being stimulated. Excess sodium may be lost, and it's important to replace it.
Q: *Where can I buy KetoStix?*
A: You can find KetoStix in any drugstore or pharmacy. For better value, try one of the shopping marts such as Costco/Price Club, Walmart, or the like.

Snack List

Smart and Delicious low carb tortilla (= 10 grams carbohydrates, Gelson's)
Mrs. May's Almond Crunch, 4 pieces (= 5 grams carbohydrates, Gelson's)
Emerald cocoa roast almonds (= 4 grams carbohydrates/minipack, Gelson's)
Blue Diamond unsweetened AlmondBreeze almondmilk (= 2 grams carbohydrates, Gelson's)
ProtiDiet oatmeal, pancake mix, cereal (= 5–7 grams carbohydrates, www.dietdirect.com)
Walden Farms jam, or other sugar free jams
Walden Farms pancake syrup
Laughing Cow Light Cheese, 2 wedges (= 1 string cheese)
Tofu shirataki noodles (whole package = 6 grams carbohydrates, Whole Foods)

Jimmy Dean low fat turkey sausage

MorningStar Farms Grilled Vegan Burger (1 patty = 7 grams carbohydrates)

Chicken gorgonzola, 1 serving (= ½ package, 9 grams carbohydrates, Trader Joe's)

Chicken pomodoro, 1 serving (= ½ package, 9 grams carbohydrates, Trader Joe's)

Tilapia citronette 1 serving (= ½ package, 6 grams carbohydrates, Trader Joe's)

THE INSULIN EXERCISE EXPERIENCE

After three days, I started an amazing
period of weight loss, consistently losing
more than 3 pounds each week. I was never
hungry, my energy level was never higher,
my blood pressure fell to 100/60, and
within three months my weight plummeted
to right where I wanted it.
—B.D., ATLANTA, GEORGIA

Do NOT skip this chapter. Even if you have no intention of doing any exercise,
please read the next few pages.

For many people the thought of exercise is so dreadful that they don't even want to read about it. They haven't done anything in the way of exercise in years and don't expect to again. The last thing a typically overweight person pictures is a vision of himself or herself working out.

Take heart! We're going to make this easy for you. In fact, the more out of shape you are, the easier it will be to benefit from the Insulin Exercise Experience.

Exercise is an integral part of the Insulin Control Diet. Without it you won't achieve the kind of success we've been promising. It's just that we recognize that the kind of exercise you need isn't the kind that first comes to mind. You won't have to start jogging or buy expensive equipment or join a gym! You will learn how to enhance your body's ability to burn fat, lose weight, and become noticeably healthier and happier, starting with just fifteen minutes per day.

The exercise program we recommend is particularly suited for those who are overweight and who haven't exercised in years or never exercised at all. Best of all, it's truly enjoyable and doesn't have to be boring. Based on our experience through the years, we're confident that you'll come to look forward to it.

But before we get down to specifics, we'd like to explain why exercise is so important for everyone interested in weight loss. We mentioned this before. Now we'll expand on it. There's more to the benefits of exercise than burning calories.

Your body contains both fat and lean muscle, but *only lean muscle is capable of burning appreciable calories.* The basic, energy-burning engine of the body is its lean muscle tissue. The fat tissue simply sits there, a storage form of energy that the body hoards. Weight reduction by diet alone can lead to large losses of lean body mass (precious protein). A person who loses considerable lean tissue is incapable of burning as many calories as before. And, when the body regains weight, it does not replace the lost muscle tissue but adds half fat and half lean tissue for each new pound. That's why it's so important to preserve precious protein.

In addition, large losses of muscle tissue can be dangerous. Not only do you lose arm and leg muscle, but you also lose critical organ muscle, especially heart muscle. As cardiac muscle is lost, the ability of the heart to function properly is compromised. That's why crash diets and extended fasting can be fatal.

The last thing you want is to lose lean tissue. You want to lose fat. That's why simply measuring the pounds you lose isn't enough. On a crash diet or when fasting, some of the weight lost is lean muscle.

Perhaps at one time or another you were a relatively lean person but exercised little. The muscle tissue you had then began to atrophy and was replaced by fat tissue. This results in less lean and more fat tissue, so you were capable of burning fewer calories daily.

Diet combined with exercise reduces the loss of precious protein and increases the burning of fat.

For a while you were in equilibrium. As your muscle tissue degenerated from lack of exercise, you added fat, but your total weight remained the same. Then slowly but surely the amount of fat increased. Even if you continued to eat only as much as before, you gained weight, and the weight brought more fat tissue. During that time, of course, there came the point when your metabolic system changed for the worse and you became insensitive to the blood sugar–lowering effects of insulin; thus you became very efficient at storing fat, not burning it.

But, you might say, you've been active all this time, working at a job or running a home. Whether you have a sedentary desk job or do work that involves physical activity, work seldom is as efficient as exercise in terms of burning calories, increasing metabolism, and building lean tissue. Regardless of how much you protest that by the end of the day you're completely exhausted, you probably have not exerted yourself in a way that is of any value so far as burning fat is concerned. Aerobic exercise is defined as activity that brings the rate of the heartbeat up significantly and keeps it there for a period of time. (We'll explain that more thoroughly in a moment.) It's only that type of exercise that achieves the goals we've been speaking of here.

HEALTH BENEFITS OF EXERCISE

A while back, dietitians and other health professionals thought that the benefit of exercise in weight loss was a matter of burning the calories coming into the body or burning off stored fat. They calculated how much of what kind of exercise it would take to burn a certain amount of calories. And, they maintained, any way you wanted to look at it, you had to burn 3,500 calories in order to lose 1 pound of fat. How discouraging to learn that even an hour of extremely strenuous activity, such as tournament-level racquetball played nonstop at top speed, would burn only 750 calories. It would take someone nearly five hours of that kind of sweating exertion to burn off just a pound of fat! And most overweight men and women are more likely to jump over the moon than to engage in that kind of physical workout.

But here's the good news. We now know that the benefits of exercise don't end when you stop exercising. Rather than merely burning the calories at the moment, your body burns many additional calories for hours afterward. After a few months of a regular exercise program, the body's metabolism undergoes a significant change and burns extra calories throughout the entire day. And, of course, the exercise builds lean tissue, which, in turn, makes your body a more effective energy-burning machine.

As you replace fat with muscle, your body can become more shapely and slender. Clothing sizes start coming down, and shopping for new, smaller clothes will be one of the rewards for following this program faithfully. When was the last time you enjoyed buying clothes?

And there are more health benefits from exercise. Several studies have now provided unequivocal evidence that regular aerobic exercise does indeed improve heart health.

Evidence of the benefits of exercising is accumulating. In one study, it was found that the risk of heart disease in university athletes directly correlated with whether these men currently or regularly exercised after they graduated. Athletes who stopped exercising after graduation were at risk, but those who continued were protected.

While most studies dealing with health and exercise have been done with men, the same benefits apply to women, along with another major advantage. Regular weight-bearing exercise has been clinically proven to reduce the risk of osteoporosis, the bone demineralizing disease we've all heard so much about in recent years. Exercise protects against osteoporosis for two reasons. First, less calcium is lost from bone tissue in those performing weight-bearing exercise. That can be as mild as regular walking. Second, calcium is better absorbed into the bones of those who exercise.

As we've seen elsewhere in this book, there's a lot of nutritional involvement with mental states. Exercise can help eliminate depression. There's a direct chemical association between exercise and mood. When you exercise, the body releases endorphins, substances that produce a soothing, happy feeling effect. The more one exercises, the more endorphins are released into the blood. When this benefit of exercise is combined with the beneficial effects on mood of the Insulin Control Diet itself, one can expect to eliminate feelings of depression and replace them with feelings of contentment.

But, you might ask, "Won't I be even hungrier when I exercise?" Actually, quite the reverse is true. Exercise tends to decrease the appetite. That's why we advocate exercise in the evening, rather than early in the morning, for those on a weight loss program. Exercise decreases blood sugar by a mechanism not involving insulin and thus decreases the need for insulin. (And, by getting out of the house, you take yourself away from the temptations of the refrigerator.)

Many overweight men and women suffer from some degree of depression.

THE EXERCISE PROGRAM

We recommend easy, regular activity. Intense exercise should be restricted during weight loss because it tends to burn glucose rather than fat. The contribution of fat as an important energy source occurs to the greatest degree at relatively mild to moderate work intensities. In the trained state, the energy requirement during exercise is increasingly met by the burning of fat. Thus, the muscle is able to spare its glycogen (animal starch reserve) for use during more demanding circumstances.

The exercise best suited for the Insulin Control Diet to help you lose weight now and keep it off forever is nothing more than walking, fine-tuned for optimum results.

Some of you may not have walked more than a city block in years. If you fear even that amount of exercise is beyond you, nothing could be further from the truth. In fact, if you are completely out of shape, it will be easier to get the activity you need to get your metabolism going in the right direction.

Many overweight people become incredibly efficient at doing little or no activity. They arrange, consciously or unconsciously, to avoid or completely eliminate movement. While watching television for the evening, they have their remote controls at hand, soft drinks close by, snacks at the ready, and telephones within easy reach. An entire evening can pass, hour after hour, without movement. For such people, simply getting off the couch and walking across the room is enough to get the heart beating rapidly. And that's exactly what we want to have happen. As we'll see, elevating the heart rate is the goal. So if you're totally out of shape, reaching that goal will be remarkably easy.

Others of you, most likely those who are in better shape, may doubt that simply walking could possibly be enough exercise to get the job done. What about the saying "No pain, no gain"? As we'll soon show you, walking can get the heart pounding for even the most athletic person.

But won't walking get boring? How can one expect to keep it up for long? Shortly, you'll find some tricks that will keep you walking for years to come. Walking can and should become a habit if done each and every day. Like any habit, this one eventually becomes hard to break.

Any form of exercise should increase your heart rate. Only when it increases well beyond the resting rate will your metabolic rate begin to change and will you begin to reap the tremendous benefits of exercise. So it's important that you understand exactly what's happening.

The heart beats at a rate sufficient to supply the entire body, including the heart itself, with oxygen-rich blood. When you're sitting still, you need less blood coursing through your arteries than when you're doing various activities. The average resting heart rate for adult men is about 72 and for women about 80. Children have a much higher rate, often about 100 beats per minute. The trained athlete may have a resting rate as low as 50. To find your own resting heart rate, simply place your forefinger on the artery to the side of your Adam's apple or at your wrist. Now count the beats for ten seconds, watching the time on a sweep-second watch. Multiply that number of beats by six and you'll have your resting heart rate in beats per minute.

If you are having difficulty measuring your heart rate, determine it by the rate of perceived exertion. For example, if you are breathing heavily and sweating (or perhaps sweating though not breathing heavily), but you can still hold a conversation, you are most likely working within your target heart rate. If you can't talk, then slow down; you are working above your target heart rate.

If you haven't been exercising regularly, don't be surprised if your resting heart rate is higher than average. This is because the heart has become inefficient at pumping enough blood to satisfy the body's needs. A strong, healthy heart can pump enough blood with little problem, requiring just a few squirts to get the blood out through the arteries. A well-trained, in-shape heart can pump a bit more blood during exercise or other activity with just a few extra beats. But the out-of-shape heart has to beat many times more. That's why when a person who has not been exercising regularly does some activity, the heart rate increases significantly.

And that brings us to your goal heart rate—the rate we'd like to have you reach during your walking sessions. Each of us has a maximum heart rate, the absolute limit of what the heart is capable of doing. Yours can be determined by subtracting your age from the number 220. It doesn't matter whether you're a man or woman, overweight or at ideal weight, or in or out of shape. If, let's say, you're forty years old, your maximum heart rate will be 220 minus 40, or 180 beats per minute.

But your heart is incapable of beating at that rate for any length of time. What you want to reach is called the training heart rate. The training rate is 80 percent of the maximum rate. For example, a forty-year-old's training heart rate will be:

$$220 - 40 = 180 \times 0.80 = 144 \text{ beats per minute}$$

Your goal in exercising is to elevate your heart rate to the training rate. However, you must reach the goal in stages. To start out, exercise to reach only 60 percent, rather than 80 percent, of maximum. For our forty-year-old this would be:

$$220 - 40 = 180 \times 0.60 = 108 \text{ beats per minute}$$

By raising your heart rate to the training level, you will begin to change your metabolism, burn fat stores more efficiently, and improve the efficiency of your heart's ability to pump blood. With only a little conditioning your resting heart rate will begin to drop. And, you will start feeling better almost immediately. That's why you don't want to put it off any longer. You don't need any special equipment, clothing, or setting. All you have to do is decide that you're going to start your Insulin Exercise Experience today.

The improvement you're going to make will be simply astounding. That's why we want you to keep an accurate record of your walking. Each day, record your resting heart rate, your heart rate while exercising, how long you walk, and a few comments about how you feel about it. (See Table 7.1.)

How long should you walk? We strongly believe that daily activity for a short period of time is infinitely better than longer, more intense activity done just once in a while. We'd like you to walk for fifteen minutes a day, every day. The best time to do so is in the evening.

Unconditioned individuals should begin at the low end of the heart rate zone and concentrate on doing long duration and low intensity at first. For example, it is strongly recommended that sedentary individuals be able to walk four miles at a brisk pace before becoming concerned with intensity. New vigorous exercisers can become easily discouraged because of muscle soreness. Starting slowly will ease the exerciser into a consistent routine. (See the recommendations in Exhibit 7.1 on page 99.)

Table 7.1 Daily Exercise Record

Date	Length of Walk	Resting Pulse	Peak Pulse	Comments (place walked, feelings, etc.)

Exhibit 7.1 Exercise Routine Recommendations by the American College of Sports Medicine (ACSM)

Warm-up: This increases circulation, heart rate, and blood pressure for more rigorous exercise and provides a smooth transition from resting exercise heart rate to higher level of activity. (Recommended: three to five minutes minimum)

Example: Choose a designated area and begin walking; walk at low intensity. Also, some light stretching is recommended. For walking, stretches should include calf muscles, shins, quadriceps (front of thigh), hamstrings (back of thigh), and ankles. Because the back is supporting you, a stretch is necessary to avoid back pain while walking.

Exercise: Twenty to sixty minutes of cardiovascular training is recommended. If you are a new exerciser, twelve to fifteen minutes of brisk exercise is sufficient. Don't worry. You can build up to twenty minutes later.

Example: Continuous brisk walking is adequate.

Cool-down: This gradually decreases heart rate to allow the body to transition back to rest.

Example: Use same routine as warm-up: light stretching and moderate movement. Heart rate should come down to 110 beats per minute within a few minutes.

Check your resting heart rate. Then start to walk at a brisk pace. How fast is fast enough? You shouldn't be able to gaze into store windows as you pass along a street. Your mind should be set on the act of walking. As you walk, you should notice your breathing increasing. You'll probably also notice a slight sheen of perspiration on your brow. But don't overdo it. While walking, you should be able to carry on a conversation without straining or sing a song without gasping for breath.

After walking along for a while, put your finger to your throat to feel the pulse in your artery. Count the beats for ten seconds as timed on your sweep-second watch. How close are you to your training heart rate? Right on target? Terrific, keep it up for the full fifteen minutes. A bit under the rate? Step up your pace. A bit faster than your training rate? Slow down. How fast you have to walk depends on what condition you're in. If you are out of shape, you may have to walk at a moderate pace so that you don't exceed your training rate. If you've been active, you may have to step right along.

Once you start getting into better shape, walking can continue to provide all the exercise you'll ever need. Simply walk a bit faster and perhaps a bit longer.

In many ways walking is superior to other kinds of exercise. Unlike jogging or running, walking is unlikely to result in any injuries. Practically every jogger will eventually succumb to shin splints, strains, sprains, stress fractures, plantar fasciitis, and other muscle and bone ailments. Unlike swimming, walking can be done at any time and any place. And there's no potential of swimmer's ear infections. Unlike aerobics, walking entails no expensive fees for classes or clubs, and there is no chance of injury associated with high-impact workouts.

Patients report time and time again that once it becomes a part of their lives, it's difficult to have to go without walking even for a single day. And, unless you're truly ill, there's no reason why you can't get those fifteen minutes of walking in daily.

Don't overdo your walking when you first begin. Ease yourself into it. Start at 60 percent of your maximum heart rate, work up to 65 percent in the first month, and don't exceed 70 percent for the first two months. Check these numbers with your doctor before you begin. If your muscles feel sore, slow down a bit. You will and should feel some muscle tension. That tension simply shows you've been doing your exercise, and it will decrease with each day of exercising. But you don't want to ache severely.

> **E**ven the most physically fit individual can reach the training heart rate with a walking program.

Regularity is the most important aspect of walking to help you lose weight. It's far better to do fifteen minutes each day than to do thirty-five or forty minutes every other day. That way one improves metabolism every day. The same applies to intensity of your exercise. It's better to maintain a steady pace than to walk so briskly that you increase the risk of tripping, pulling a muscle, or wearing yourself out so that you have to stop. If you feel after a few weeks that you're ready for more exercise, simply increase the amount of time you spend walking each day. Go from fifteen minutes to twenty to thirty and so on.

When you're in better shape and walking fifteen to thirty minutes every day, you may find that you can no longer reach your target training heart rate in that thirty minutes. If you have the time and inclination, you can simply walk longer distances over a longer period of time. However, if the time you have available for exercise is limited, you can increase the difficulty of your walks in order to use your limited time more efficiently. Here are a couple of suggestion to get your heart rate up faster.

First, hand weights will increase the amount of work you do while walking and you'll find your heart rate increasing. Don't overdo it. Start with the smallest weight you can find and gradually build up. The last thing you want to do is to hurt yourself.

Second, pick up a small knapsack. Place a 5-pound bag of sugar or flour in it, and walk with that amount of weight for a week. Gradually increase the weight as you're able to do so while staying within your training heart rate zone.

For most people this increase in workload will not be necessary. You'll get the results you want if you just continue to do your fifteen minutes of walking each day. Remember that the most important part of this exercise experience is consistency. Once you've gotten into the routine of daily exercise, try increasing the amount you do. Instead of fifteen minutes, walk for twenty minutes, then twenty-five, and then thirty. Next, try to get out not just once, but twice daily. Or, if your schedule doesn't permit that, try walking once a day and doing some other exercise some other time during the day.

ENJOYING YOUR WALKING EXPERIENCE

After just the first two or three weeks, you'll start to realize that you won't want to give up walking. Perhaps you'll want to treat yourself to a new pair of walking shoes. A number of high-quality shoes specifically designed for walking are on the market. They look like jogging shoes, but the soles are more flexible and have less cushioning than the soles designed to soften the impact of running. Shop around for a pair that feels particularly comfortable for you.

You can walk alone or with friends. You can walk through a park, along a crowded avenue, or in an indoor shopping mall. You could not be getting into this activity at a better time. Walking clubs are starting up all over the country. (To find clubs in your area you might contact the American Volkssports Association, 1001 Pat Booker Road, Universal City, Texas 78148, or visit the organization's website, http://ava.org.)

To make your walking experience as enjoyable as possible, we've developed a series of suggestions to keep you interested and looking forward to the next outing. Your personal schedule will determine when you'll be able to do the various suggested walks. If you can, plan two or three days ahead, so you'll have something to look forward to.

Remember that your main purpose is to walk for the exercise. Make sure that you do your full fifteen minutes of walking without stopping to look in shop windows or smell the roses in the park. After you've done your vigorous walking, you may wish to stroll through the park or window-shop. But never forget that the two types of walking are different in their purposes.

The most convenient walk is around your block. It's probably the best way to start, and there will be days when it's all you'll have time to do. As you start out, time how long it takes you to walk a block and calculate how many blocks you'll be able to walk at your training heart rate during your fifteen minutes. Then map out other routes.

Some days you may wish to get into your car and drive a mile or so away to take your walk. Pick up a street map of your area. Map out the areas you want to walk in, and assign yourself different chunks of your town or city for different days. Soon you'll know the city better than any cab driver! If you live in a rural area, the same principles apply. Does your city have a Chinatown or other ethnic areas? How many parks do you have in your community? Try to do walking tours of each of them. Relive a part of the history of your area by imagining yourself living during an earlier time, walking, say, the route of Paul Revere.

On rainy or extremely cold days, find an indoor shopping mall where you can really stretch your legs. Some of the new ones have two or three levels, and you can really work up a good sweat in fifteen minutes. Many malls open their doors before business hours so that walkers can take an indoor hike before shoppers crowd the lanes. And after your walk, give yourself a little reward such as a nice hot cup of tea.

Sedentary people are more likely to experience the difficulties associated with aging.

Make a list of the places you'd like to go walking. In many cities, your list can include museums, zoos, plant conservatories, boardwalks, and various public buildings. After your walk, put your comments into your daily exercise record. Was it a walk you want to repeat? How did it rate on a scale of 1 to 10?

STRETCHING EXERCISES

We'd like to encourage you to do some simple stretching exercises that will enhance your total program of weight loss and toning. The stretches we've selected are soothing and will gradually increase your flexibility. Do them immediately after your walk each day. Do as much as you can without straining. As time goes on, you'll find that you're able to stretch farther and farther.

By increasing your flexibility at the same time you build up your stamina and lose weight, you'll be at much less risk of the injuries that so often accompany the aging process.

Do these stretches in the order given. Hold each stretch for one count at first, and then work up to a count of ten. Stretch only to the point of feeling the stretch, not to the point of pain. Relax and *breathe*.

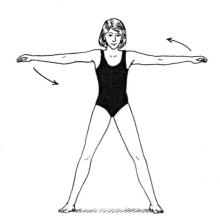

1. Stand straight and lift your arms out to the sides. Turn the upper torso to one side. Count while feeling the tension. Repeat to the other side. Keep knees soft and stomach pulled in.

2. Stand straight. Use a chair or the wall for balance. Bend one leg up to the back and grasp your ankle. Gently pull your leg toward your body and count. Repeat with the other leg. If walking outdoors, you can use a park bench, anything to keep your balance.

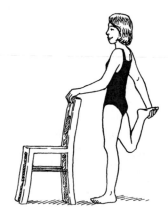

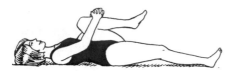

3. In either a standing or reclining position, pull one knee to your chest. Count. Repeat with the other leg. Soften opposite leg if you have back trouble, but do not straighten.

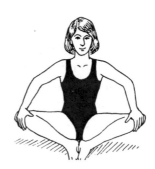

4. Sit on the floor and bring both feet into the groin. Gently push your knees as close to the floor as possible. Sit upright. Count.

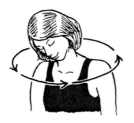

5. While comfortably seated, slightly look to the right and follow to the left. Do this slowly! Hold for ten to thirty seconds on each side. Option: Tilt ear to shoulder and hold for ten to thirty seconds. Do not press or pull the head. Avoid overstretching. You may take the chin to the chest. *Do not bring head backward.*

6. Stand upright and place your hands on a wall or a sturdy support. Extend one leg to the rear. Bend the other knee, pressing the heel of the extended foot downward to exert stretch on calf. Count. Repeat for other leg. You may bend the extended leg slightly at the knee to stretch the soleus muscles (below the belly of the calf muscle).

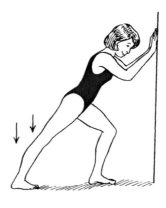

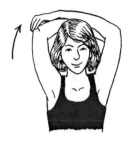

7. Stand upright. Attempt to touch the center of your back by reaching over your shoulder. Assist with your other hand by pulling gently on your elbow. Count. Repeat with the other arm.

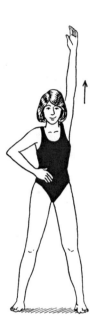

8. Stand upright. Attempt to touch the ceiling with each hand alternately; then both together for a count of ten each. Soften the knees, and hold in your stomach. Elderly or severely overweight individuals can do this exercise while sitting down.

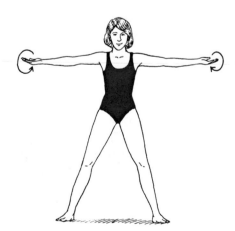

9. Stand upright, and lift your arms out to the sides. Extend your arms as far as possible. With palms up, circle arms to the back ten times. Circle to the front ten times. Repeat with palms down. Soften your knees, and hold in your stomach.

10. Stand upright. Let your right hand slide down your right leg as your left hand reaches for the ceiling. Bend the torso toward the right, keeping shoulders straight forward and arm stretched. Count. Repeat on the opposite side. Soften your knees, and hold in your stomach. Elderly or severely overweight persons can sit in a chair during this exercise.

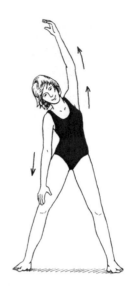

Relaxing After Exercise

We strongly recommend you lie down and relax after completing your exercise. This will allow the body to release fluids stored during that exercise period. Following your rest you will probably feel the need to urinate.

Let us explain a bit of the way the body works along these lines. The kidneys are pressure pumps, needing more of the heart's output of blood than any other organ in the body to excrete their quota of fluid for the day. Particularly in women, vigorous exercise tends to shunt blood away from the kidneys to the exercising muscle, resulting in less water loss than would have occurred at rest.

But you don't want that fluid stored. Taking a rest after the exercise period allows that water to be released.

OTHER EXERCISE POSSIBILITIES

While we believe walking is the best possible form of exercise, ultimately the best is the exercise you will be most likely to continue indefinitely. You may prefer to do some other activity, or you may want to alternate exercise activities. And there will be times when walking is out of the question due to bad weather.

Swimming is an excellent form of exercise. As with any activity, start with a few laps and gradually build up to longer total distances. Does your YMCA/YWCA have aquatic exercise in the pool? That is a growing and enjoyable method of good exercise.

Stationary bicycles are excellent for working your heart up to the target rate. You can buy one or use one at a local YMCA/YWCA or health club. (If you do decide to buy, two brands known for high quality are Tunturi and Schwinn.)

Other apparatuses are not as efficient and look better in principle than in action. And some may be harder on the back or other parts of the body. Investigate potential benefits and harm of any given machine before buying.

Again, the best exercise is the exercise that you *do* on a regular basis.

EXERCISE FOR A LIFETIME

Although you probably can't imagine it now, as time goes on you'll not only be able to increase your exercise, but you will actually want to do so. Although Hippocrates used more formal wording, his recommendation hundreds of years ago remains valid today: Use it or lose it! We all want to remain vibrant, active, and healthy for a good quality of life as well as quantity of life.

Plan on exercising three to five times per week; three times is the minimum. Do so for twenty to sixty minutes of continuous exercise; twenty minutes is the minimum. Based on your heart rate, you'll want to exercise at 60 percent to 90 percent of your maximum heart rate.

Bear in mind, though, that these are considerations for the future. Right now it's perfectly adequate to simply do a nice walk, as briskly as you can without overexertion, fifteen to twenty minutes every day. Remember the Chinese proverb: The journey of a thousand miles begins with a single step.

Thank you for reading this chapter. If you're still skeptical about exercising, even in the easygoing and pleasant ways described, give it a try. Do the walking and the stretching for just a month. You certainly can do that. It's only a month, and what have you got to lose? We're absolutely positive that after a month you'll never want to quit. The Insulin Exercise Experience will become a part of your life.

Chapter 8

STABILIZATION

*For me this is far more than a diet book. It
is a concept, a system of reasonable, easy-to-
assume habits for wholesome, healthy, and
comfortable living. One of the book's more
delightful effects is the growing awareness
that you are referring to it less and less as
the program becomes part of your life.*
—S.B., Tucson, Arizona

Congratulations! You've shed those pounds and inches and
attained your desired goal weight. You have complied with our
guidelines for food consumption and restriction. You have entered a
program of regular exercise and are doing some form of physical
activity every day. You've kept a detailed diary of everything you ate
and drank and all the exercise you've done. It's been an effort, but
it's been worth it, and now you want to make sure you never gain
that weight back again.

Your success in stabilization will require a continued commitment. It's best to go along with our diet recommendations as strictly
as you can. It's essential to continue your exercise program; ideally,
you should exercise daily, with at least twenty to thirty minutes of
walking, bicycle riding, or indoor aerobic activity. By all means continue to keep your daily diary. The odds for successful stabilization
and maintenance favor those who follow these three suggestions.

But before you begin to stabilize at your current weight, be certain that this is the weight at which you really want to live the rest
of your life. Too often dieters decide it's time to stop before they
reach their goal weights. Some look in the mirror and say what they
see is good enough. Others aren't really satisfied but decide to accept

a compromise. Still others are persuaded by well-meaning friends and relatives that they should stop dieting.

Early in the program, after initial success, you will have the confidence to set a goal weight. If it is a realistic goal, then don't be persuaded to give up early. People who achieve their goal weights are much more likely to maintain their weight loss permanently. Discuss your goal weight with your physician to determine the weight best for you. For those who have a family history of Type 2 diabetes, a lower goal weight is more effective in diabetes prevention.

Remember, there's no mystery in this. If you settle now for a weight that's, let's say, 10 or 15 pounds above your original goal, you'll not find it too difficult to accept just another pound or two. Then the next month it will be OK to add another pound or two. And before you know it, you've gained all that lost weight back—and perhaps even more than you started with.

So give this a great deal of thought before you leave ketosis and begin to stabilize. Be absolutely certain that you weigh what you want to weigh and that you've achieved your goal.

> **R**emember, the less fat you carry the less insulin resistance remains.

Perhaps when you began this diet you doubted the idea of limiting your carbohydrate intake so severely. You might have thought that it wouldn't really be necessary to follow the guidelines rigidly. Then you found that in order to stay in ketosis, carbohydrate intake did indeed have to be kept way down and that deviation from the guidelines took you out of ketosis.

Remember this as you enter the period of stabilization. Again, these guidelines have been proven time and again to be the most effective way to deal with this process. Stay within these guidelines, and you'll succeed beautifully.

PROCESS OF STABILIZATION

To understand the process of stabilization, think of your body as a beaker in which you, a chemist, are trying to create just the right solution. You will have the right solution when it turns from yellow to green. You add one chemical into another chemical already in the beaker just one drop at a time so that you can measure exactly how much of the first chemical it really takes to get the job done. Finally, one more drop in a long series is the one to complete the reaction and make the color change. If you had simply dumped a lot of the chemical in at once, the color change would have occurred, but you'd never know how much more was added than necessary. In science this process of gradual adding is called titration.

To stabilize your weight so that you neither lose nor gain, you have to determine exactly how much food and what kinds of food you can add to your diet. You know that the diet you're currently following causes you to lose weight, but now you've lost enough. Just how much more can you eat before you stop losing weight and before you begin to gain weight? No one knows. Each person is different, and there's no formula that will tell you the exact number of calories and grams of carbohydrates needed to stabilize and maintain your weight. So we titrate; that is, we add food little by little to measure accurately how much and what kind causes a reaction.

During the weight loss phase, you have been feeding yourself in two ways. First, your food has provided 1,000 to 1,500 calories. Second, you have received at least 1,000 additional calories from your stored fat, which has been converted to energy.

To stop losing weight you must now begin to increase your food, and thus your caloric intake. You'll do this gradually with a combination of complex carbohydrates and monounsaturated fats added to your present protein intake.

Weight loss produces a decrease in metabolism, a phenomenon that probably evolved to ensure survival during times of famine. As you increase your calories taken as food, metabolism increases by favoring the production of the active form of the thyroid hormone.

Ultimately, if you are burning 2,000 calories daily, you will have to consume that number of calories to maintain a constant ideal weight. That number will vary, of course, depending upon your level of physical activity and your individual body stature. Remember that the more lean muscle tissue you have, the more calories can be burned.

How should your caloric allowance be divided into fat, proteins, and carbohydrates? No more than 30 percent of the day's calories should come from fat, with the emphasis placed on monounsaturated fats from foods such as olive and canola oils, and avoiding saturated fats from animal foods and tropical oils. That means, for a person consuming 2,000 calories, 600 calories will come from fat. Since fat has 9 calories per gram, that means one's daily fat allotment would be 66 grams.

Next we calculate 50 percent of calories from carbohydrates. Again, for the person requiring 2,000 calories daily, that means 1,000 of those calories will come from carbohydrates. And because carbohydrates provide 4 calories per gram, that person will consume about 250 grams of carbohydrates.

That leaves 20 percent of our daily calories, which will be derived from proteins. For the person consuming 2,000 calories, this will mean 400 protein calories. Like carbohydrates, protein provides 4 calories per gram; therefore, 100 grams will yield those 400 calories.

Of course, you won't jump directly to 2,000 calories or any other predetermined number. Rather, you will gradually add calories until you no longer lose—nor gain—weight. Perhaps you'll reach 2,000 calories. Perhaps the number will be greater or less. Regardless of the total, however, the percentage will remain the same: 30 percent as fat, 50 percent as carbohydrate, and 20 percent as protein. For diabetics the carbohydrate allowance may have to be substantially reduced in favor of more "good" fats to maintain normal blood sugars.

Bear in mind the concept of titration and the need to find exactly the right caloric intake. But it's also true that those added carbohydrates may trigger salt and water retention. This may be aggravated by vigorous exercise, which diverts blood away from the kidneys.

Deal with this dilemma by returning temporarily to ketosis and utilizing the concept of the diuresis of recumbency. When weight has returned to goal level, you can once again add back the carbohydrate, but perhaps in smaller increments.

Don't be dismayed if during the stabilization period you begin to gain weight.

THYROID HORMONE AND THE STARVATION WEIGHT MODE

Thyroid hormone produced by your body's thyroid gland in the neck plays a large role in metabolism. It exerts its influence as one form, thyroxine (T4), is converted to triiodothyronine (T3) by way of an enzyme that is sensitive to carbohydrate. When there is less carbohydrate available, less T4 will be converted to T3, and metabolism is decreased. This is the mechanism by which the body conserves its energy in times of famine and starvation.

This has practical implications for you when following the Insulin Control Diet, because as metabolism decreases, the body produces less heat and you may feel cold. The answer to this problem is an increase in exercise. As always, this does not mean strenuous aerobics. Rather, a slight increase in physical activity will communicate the need to step up the metabolism. Try taking an additional one-mile walk, for example. Your metabolism will increase, and you'll feel warmer.

During the stabilization phase, you'll gradually add back some carbohydrate, which will directly influence the T4/T3 conversion. Again, the emphasis is on small, stepwise, incremental increases.

Marching Through Stabilization

In the first week of stabilization, you add 5 grams of carbohydrate and 1 ounce of protein food to your daily meal plan. For example, instead of 4 ounces of chicken at lunch, make it 5. Or add another ounce of fish to your evening meal. The choice of carbohydrates is yours, but make your carbohydrate selections from the vegetable list during that first week. Perhaps it will be half a cup of green beans, broccoli, or cauliflower with your evening meal. Maybe you'd like to nibble on half an artichoke during the evening. Or you might opt for a 4-ounce glass of tomato juice before a meal or in the afternoon.

Assuming that you're continuing your program of exercise, you may lose another pound or two during that first week of stabilization. In fact, you probably will. Depending on the amount of physical activity that now marks each day, you may even lose more than that. But that's just fine, because you'll be adding foods gradually.

Add another ounce of protein and another 5 grams of carbohydrate during the second week and again during the third week. During the fourth week of stabilization, you will add a final ounce of protein to reach a full 13 to 15 ounces daily. How you divide your portions depends on your own preferences. Would you like to have a larger breakfast, with a piece of meat added to your egg? Do you prefer to have a larger portion of meat with your evening meal? The 13 to 15 ounces, however, is the maximum allotted protein throughout stabilization and as you maintain your weight for years to come.

This amount of protein, coming from meat, fish, poultry, cheese, and eggs, will more than satisfy your body's requirements. In fact, the total amount of protein will be larger than the Recommended Reference Intakes. No man or woman needs more, regardless of physical activity.

But, again depending on your energy output as determined by the amount of exercise you're now doing, you very well may need more calories. So, during the fourth and fifth weeks of stabilization you'll add one daily carbohydrate serving.

This is the time to stress the utmost importance of eating a variety of foods. Every nutrition authority agrees with the value of such variety from the food groups. The Japanese government urges its citizens to eat thirty-five different kinds of food each day. Of course, portions would be small, as in a salad or a stew containing many different ingredients.

Additional calories during stabilization may also come from fat. As always, diabetic individuals should avoid saturated fats even more stringently than the general population because of the increased risk of heart disease. Monounsaturated fats, however, do not raise cholesterol levels and may be used interchangeably with carbohydrates in adding calories.

Remember that *all* fats add 9 calories per gram, as compared with 4 calories per gram of either protein or carbohydrate. Sources of monounsaturated fat include olive and canola oils, olives, avocados, and cashews.

The added carbohydrates will come from fruit, vegetables, breads, cereals, and pasta. You may decide to add fruit by having a larger piece instead of adding another kind; instead of a half pear, you may want a whole one.

We've neglected one food group until now—the milk group. You may now feel free to have a glass of skim milk or a serving of nonfat or low fat yogurt. Certainly these dairy foods provide enjoyment and nutrients, but since the calcium supplement you now take will provide all the calcium you need, there isn't a strict nutritional reason for consuming dairy foods. If you wish, enjoy a serving of nonfat milk or yogurt during the fifth week of stabilization. This will be *in place* of both a serving of carbohydrate and a serving of protein, since milk and yogurt contain both. You must also be aware of any flavorings in the yogurt; most have added sugar and fruit that boost the carbohydrate level considerably.

By the end of the fifth week of stabilization, you will be consuming a wide variety of foods from all the food groups. The number of servings will depend entirely upon your own individual metabolism.

The stabilization process should take at least four to five weeks of gradually adding carbohydrates and protein until you reach a point of balance. Don't try to rush the process by adding two carbohydrate servings at a time. Keep that cautious chemist in mind, titrating according to your special, individual needs.

As you proceed, you'll want to keep accurate records in your diet diary. Those who add foods systematically and record those foods faithfully are far more likely to succeed.

> The stabilization process should take at least four weeks of gradually adding carbohydrates and protein until you reach a point of balance.

How much carbohydrate will you be able to add to your diet? There's no way to predict the total, other than in relation to the amount of your lean muscle mass, your level of physical activity, and the control of your blood sugar. Larger individuals, with bigger bones and more substantial muscles, will undoubtedly be able to consume more carbohydrate than smaller individuals. On the other hand, smaller people who exercise a lot may be able to eat as much as larger, sedentary individuals. But there are unfortunate and unexpected exceptions to the basic rules of thumb. There are large, active men who find they can add very little carbohydrate. And there are small women who, once they lose fat tissue, are able to consume quite a bit. Some men and women will be able to go up to only 75 grams of carbohydrates daily, others up to 250 grams. Some diabetics will have difficulty with even a little more carbohydrate than they consumed on the weight loss program, and they may require medication to control their blood sugars.

Thus far we've talked only about adding foods to the diet. There may be times when you have to subtract some. If, after two or three weeks of stabilization, you find that you're starting to gain a bit of weight, cut back on the carbohydrates. A week later try the additional carbohydrate again, and see if you gain. If you do not, continue with that amount for another week before trying the next carbohydrate increase. If you're still not gaining, go on from there.

You may go all the way through four or five weeks of stabilization without gaining a pound, only to have a sudden weight surge. This is where your food diary and exercise record will come in handy. Read them carefully. Perhaps you upped the carbohydrate intake beyond what you thought it was. Perhaps your exercise program suffered a bit owing to a slight cold. Perhaps you ate in a restaurant and did not know what all the ingredients were in the meal. Try to eliminate such variables, and see if the weight gain continues. If it does, you'll have to subtract one of the carbohydrates, perhaps going back to half a pear rather than a whole one for a snack. Or, you can increase your exercise. Do an extra hour of walking for the week. Get in another bicycle ride. Take another aerobics class. Work that metabolism up to where you can consume that additional food without weight gain.

SIMPLE SUGARS: STILL THE NUMBER ONE POISON

One person may be able to add carbohydrates and proteins to the diet every week throughout stabilization without gaining an ounce. Another individual may find that only one or two servings of carbohydrates can be added without weight gain. Certainly there are distinct genetic differences among men and women that we have no control over. The amount of lean muscle mass will also determine the level of energy that can be burned efficiently. And, of course, the time spent in rigorous physical activity directly correlates with just how much total food, including carbohydrates, can be eaten without weight gain.

The one food that almost everyone who has had a weight problem will have difficulty with is simple sugar. Whether in the guise of a candy bar, a piece of cake, pasta, a slice of pie, or a bowl of sweetened cereal, simple sugars remain the Number One Poison for most people, even after they've lost weight and begun a regular program of exercise. Avoid them whenever possible. For some people this is easier than for others. For one patient, Margaret, staying away from sugar also prevented the headaches she had suffered for years without knowing the source of her pain. Just a small serving was enough to bring on throbbing pain. So she never ate enough to return her to the metabolic trap.

Concentrate on the many, many foods you can enjoy without the fear of regaining the pounds and inches you successfully shed. Whether it's a main meal or a midday snack, there are many choices available to you without dipping into foods laden with sugars. Do you *really* want to risk weight gain for the small and transient pleasure of a piece of candy? Practically everyone has to come to grips with avoiding one pleasure or another for the sake of health and well-being.

For the person who quits smoking cigarettes, we know that having "just a puff" now and then or "just one" cigarette after a nice Saturday evening dinner is flirting with disaster. Certainly there is the temptation to start thinking that one no longer is addicted to tobacco and thus can enjoy that occasional smoke. But the truth is harsh and simple. The only way to stay away from the habit is to eliminate smoking completely from one's life.

On the positive side, former smokers will tell you that the times when one craves a cigarette grow more and more infrequent and the craving, when it does strike, becomes less and less intense as time goes on. The habit *can* be kicked for good.

And the same applies to simple sugars. Having been a victim of the metabolic trap, your body is far more vulnerable to the horrors of insulin resistance than others. Even though you are slender at this point, insulin levels can soar with just the smallest slice of pie or piece of cake. We wish it weren't so, but it's simply a physiological fact of life that you'll have to deal with now and forever.

To cite another analogy, many authorities now believe that alcoholism is a disease that can be genetically determined and that has little if anything to do with a person's willpower or self-control. The body of an alcoholic reacts differently to ingestion of alcohol than does the body of a social drinker, who can consume alcoholic beverages moderately for years without dependence. When the alcoholic determines to stay sober, he or she must accept the truth that even one drink is too much. It must be total abstinence for life. That's why groups refer to the sober drinker as a "recovering" rather than a "recovered" alcoholic. The disease is always there, ready to return at the first indiscretion.

It's interesting to realize, then, that there are alcoholics who have never had a drink in their lives. Alcoholism is a disease that requires a stimulus, namely, alcohol, to make itself manifest. Therefore, if one is born an alcoholic by genetic potential and a member of a non-drinking religious sect such as the Mormons or the Seventh-Day Adventists, one will never exhibit the inability to consume alcohol in moderation. And that, certainly, is a blessing.

The same can be said for those genetically determined to become noninsulin-dependent diabetics. Without the factor of overweight, the diabetes may never become manifest. Conversely, if a diabetic patient successfully loses the weight, symptoms of diabetes frequently completely disappear. Does that mean the diabetic has been "cured"? Not really, since the disease is ready to reappear if weight is regained.

For the alcoholic, no drink should be worth the degradation alcohol can cause. And for the formerly overweight man or woman, simple sugars, the Number One Poison, are simply not worth the return to a state of obesity. Unlike former smokers and recovering alcoholics, however, there are some now-slender dieters who can enjoy an occasional special treat. Some can take a taste of dessert and leave the rest behind. Are you one of these? Can you have just *one bite* of cake? Just one small piece of candy? Just one cookie? For some the little taste is satisfying; for others it's self-inflicted torture to be tantalized with a taste only to have the urge to gorge denied.

You may decide on occasion to say "the hell with it" and enjoy yourself with a food you shouldn't have, knowing full well that in the morning you'll have gained weight. You'll have to weigh the risks and benefits. But if you do "fall off the wagon" at a special meal or just for the pleasure of a hot fudge sundae, you have to do so with your eyes wide-open. Accept that you probably will gain some weight. But also anticipate that you'll go right back to your healthful diet.

The real danger in this situation is the temptation to say, "Well, I've gained a pound, so if I gain another pound today it won't be too bad." That kind of thinking can lead one right back to obesity and the metabolic trap.

Another, probably safer, approach might be to anticipate an occasion where you'll want to splurge. Let's say you're invited to a party on Saturday evening, and you'll want to join the other guests in eating dessert. Knowing this in advance, you can "save up" for the party by avoiding carbohydrates all day Friday and Saturday until dinner. Perhaps you may also need to eliminate starch on Sunday as well to make up for your indulgence. But you will be able to enjoy that special treat.

As time goes on, most formerly overweight men and women come to accept their dietary limitations, rather like the smoker who, after a while, seldom thinks about having a cigarette. By avoiding the simple sugars as much as possible, you'll find it easier to achieve that state of mind. Ultimately, only you will be able to find out what works best for you and make your own decisions.

A NEW IMAGE

As you progress through your period of stabilization, concentrate on a new self-image. You are no longer an overweight person. Believe it or not, in one way or another, you've gotten used to the idea of being heavy. You may even have used it as an excuse for doing one thing or not doing another. Now it's time to make an entirely new life for yourself as a slender person.

Look in the mirror and allow yourself to enjoy what you see. Take pride in your achievement, for which you alone can take all of the credit. Say it right out loud: "I *love* myself, and I *love* my new body." Now prove it by being nice to yourself. You deserve the reward for your effort.

This is the time to read Chapter 10 on support again. Think again about the important lifestyle changes you must make in order to be slim for the rest of your life. You've lost the weight you wanted to lose; the period of stabilization is critical if you want to keep it off.

This is the time to take charge of your life, and enjoy it to the fullest.

It's important to start thinking of yourself as a thin person. How is a slender person different from the way you were before you lost weight? Slender people seem to have more energy and be more active. You've probably noticed those traits in yourself lately; now believe they are real changes and capitalize on them. Slender men and women enjoy their meals without overeating. Many people who have weight problems tend to look and act with little confidence; try being a bit more assertive.

In the past you may have thought of yourself as a thin person in a fat body. Now perhaps you're beginning to feel like a fat person in a thin body. Think of the things you wanted to do when you were heavy but were unable to do. This is the time to take charge of your life and enjoy it to the fullest.

It's sometimes helpful to take some snapshots of yourself today and compare them with those taken when you were overweight. Look at the difference. Convince yourself that you really are slender and that it's worth all your efforts to remain that way.

Exercise may have been quite a chore when you first started the program. As you became used to it, physical activity became easier. Now that you're slender, exercise has probably become an important, positive pleasure in your life. Enjoy the way your body responds to your commands for movement. You glide across the room in comparison to the way you moved in the past; your walking stride has grace. You can feel your muscles flex and enjoy touching the firmness of your body.

Get used to the compliments you're hearing on your new slender appearance. Don't be embarrassed by them. When you receive a compliment, you can honestly respond, "Thanks. I feel much better, too!"

Never, never let anyone convince you that you're too thin if you feel great at your present weight, especially if that's the weight your doctor recommends. Friends and relatives may try to convince you that you looked better with "just a bit more weight" or that some people are simply meant to be on the heavy side. There are reasons why our loved ones may not be pleased with our weight loss. Change can be threatening to others. Eating and drinking love company, and our abstinence and self-control may make others uncomfortable. Competitiveness and jealousy might even be motivations. The misconception that more flesh on the bones means more robust health may still hold sway with some people.

On the other hand, if everyone seems to be telling you that you're too thin and losing too much weight, it makes sense to evaluate those concerns seriously and honestly. Do you perceive yourself as you really are? Are you maintaining your low weight by practically starving yourself or making yourself miserable and nervous? Do you feel healthy? If you can satisfy yourself on these counts, stick to your guns. Tell them some people might be meant to be on the heavy side, but you're not one of them—and never will be again.

After five—or up to six or even eight—weeks, you will have stabilized your weight. This is the beginning of the maintenance phase. That's another phase for the rest of your life.

STABILIZATION AT A GLANCE

Week One

- Weigh yourself daily.
- Maintain your dietary diary and exercise record.
- Add one vegetable carbohydrate serving to your current daily diet.
- Add 1 ounce of protein to your current daily diet (a total of 9 ounces for women, 11 ounces for men).
- Maintain daily exercise.
- Consume eight 8-ounce glasses of fluid daily.

Week Two

- Weigh yourself daily.
- Maintain your dietary diary and exercise record.
- If you have not gained or lost weight during the first week, add another vegetable carbohydrate. If you have lost weight, add one fruit carbohydrate.
- Add 1 ounce of protein (a total of 10 ounces for women, 12 ounces for men).
- Try to exercise one hour daily.
- Consume eight 8-ounce glasses of fluid daily.
- Work on your image of your new, slender self.

Week Three

- Weigh yourself daily.
- Maintain your dietary diary and exercise record.
- If you wish, you may add 1 more ounce of protein (a total of 11 ounces for women, 13 ounces for men). Choose lean cuts of meat, white meat poultry, and fish.
- If you are still losing weight, add two servings of carbohydrate. These can be fruit, vegetable, or bread.
- If you are maintaining your weight, add one carbohydrate serving of your choice.
- Consume eight 8-ounce glasses of fluid daily.
- *Avoid simple sugars!*

Week Four

- Weigh yourself daily.
- Maintain your dietary diary and exercise record.
- Add another ounce of protein, if desired.
- You may now be approaching your maximum carbohydrate intake potential. Add one carbohydrate serving. If you gain weight, eliminate it.
- If you're not gaining weight, you may now add 1 teaspoon of oil to your daily diet.
- Continue to exercise daily.
- Consume eight 8-ounce glasses of fluid daily.

Week Five

- Weigh yourself daily.
- Maintain your dietary diary and exercise record.
- Only if you are now exercising extensively and feel that you can afford the added calories, add one more carbohydrate to your diet. Watch the scale carefully each day to be sure you don't gain any weight.
- If you wish, you may now have a glass of nonfat milk or a cup of nonfat yogurt in place of 1 ounce of protein and 1 carbohydrate.
- Consume eight 8-ounce glasses of fluid daily.

• At this point you are consuming a totally balanced diet and are able to consume all foods except simple sugars.

Week Six

• Weigh yourself daily.
• Maintain your dietary diary and exercise record.
• If your weight continues to fluctuate, carefully analyze your diary to determine what may be causing the weight gain or loss. Check your (1) exercise, (2) simple sugar consumption, (3) fat consumption, (4) fruit carbohydrate consumption, and (5) total caloric intake. Adjust your daily diet as necessary. You may increase your exercise activity if you need to burn more calories.
• Consume eight 8-ounce glasses of fluid daily.

Week Seven and Forever

• Weigh yourself every other day.
• Add or subtract foods as needed to maintain weight.
• Maintain an energetic daily exercise regimen of brisk walking, bicycle riding, sports, or aerobics.
• Consume eight 8-ounce glasses of fluid daily.
• Practice relaxation techniques (Chapter 10) and improve your self-image.
• Enjoy your slender body and give yourself credit for your success!

Chapter 9

MAINTAINING WEIGHT LOSS PERMANENTLY

*During the past four and a half months, I
have lost 35 pounds and I have my diabetes
under control. I feel 100 percent better,
have more energy, and I do not tire as
quickly as I did before. My blood tests have
returned to normal.*
—R.P., NORTH HILLS, CALIFORNIA

Probably for the first time in your life, you have a good grasp of how your body works. You know just how much food you can eat daily without gaining or losing weight. You're feeling better because of your exercise program, and you're more in tune with your body. You're sleeping better at night, with increased daytime energy, and have control of carbohydrate cravings, all from the assistance of trazodone. You feel a strong sense of satisfaction, knowing that you've done something worthwhile in losing weight. It may well be that you've never felt better in your life. Now's the time to make a promise to yourself that this is the way you're going to feel for the rest of your life.

It is not true that everyone who ever lost weight with this program kept it off. But we can say that everyone who succeeded made a commitment to a lifetime of loving himself or herself enough to really care about his or her own well-being. It's up to you to make that commitment to yourself, to be absolutely certain that you won't harm yourself by regaining those pounds and inches. You now have the knowledge to make it all work, and Chapter 10 will give you new skills that you can use when you need to bolster your resolve.

Why is it far more difficult to sustain weight loss than to achieve it? Most individuals who lose weight gain it back. This can be explained by the more drastic reduction of insulin that accompanies weight loss rather than weight maintenance, in addition to the depletion of serotonin from the stress of dieting. Lack of serotonin produces carbohydrate cravings and daytime fatigue. (For more details see the Doctor to Doctor chapter.) Therefore, weight maintenance must be considered a lifelong effort.

Long before you fell into the metabolic trap that made you virtually helpless to lose weight, you began to gain weight slowly but surely. Regardless of the circumstances—and everyone has his or her own story to tell—that weight gain at the beginning was due to a surplus of calories and a deficit of physical activity, with disturbed sleep from stress-induced depletion of serotonin. Only after you gained a significant amount of weight did your insulin-induced carbohydrate addiction join the enemy team to add to the pounds and inches. Once that happened, of course, you were out of control and almost any diet or program would have ended in failure.

But that's all changed now. You've escaped the metabolic trap, and there's no reason to fall into it again. Massive weight gain begins with the gain of just a single pound. There are two ways you can make sure you don't put on that pound.

First, throughout the maintenance phase you can continue with the program for the last week of stabilization. Count the servings of protein and carbohydrates you eat each day, drink adequate water, exercise regularly, and weigh yourself every other day to make sure you haven't regained. This approach has worked for hundreds of men and women. You know it has worked thus far for you, and it can continue to do so forever.

Second, you can take the dietary approach that most medical and nutrition authorities agree is the ultimate way to maintain desired weight permanently and at the same time postpone the onset of degenerative disease and enhance longevity. Many people lose weight without even trying to do so when they change their diets to improve their health.

The recommendation for a longer, healthier life is unequivocal—eat less fat, especially less saturated fat, and less cholesterol. By focusing on low fat intake, you may achieve two goals: maintaining ideal weight (without counting calories) and attaining optimal health.

Maintaining desired weight comes down to giving your body just enough food to support itself. Feed the body you want to have. If you give a 150-pound body enough food to feed a 200-pound body, predictably you'll have a 200-pound body. And, if you give a 200-pound body just enough food to feed a 150-pound body, you'll have a 150-pound body. But weight loss is not quite that simple, as you've learned through the years. When you stop feeding that 200-pound body, providing only enough for 150 pounds, the other 50 pounds start screaming: Feed me! Feed me! The challenge is to hold out long enough to make those 50 pounds disappear. And, as we now know so well, the influence of the metabolic trap with increased insulin and decreased serotonin makes the weight loss nearly impossible. If the weight loss you had to deal with originally was even more than 50 pounds, the odds against your success were astronomical.

> Just as simple sugar is the Number One Poison for those caught in the metabolic trap, fat is the Number One Killer when it comes to degenerative diseases, including heart disease and cancer.

But now, through this program, you've wiped the slate clean and are starting out again. You do weigh 150 pounds or 120 pounds or whatever your desired goal weight is. You can now learn to feed only those desired pounds. You may say that you've tried counting calories before and that can be a dismal and frustrating way to live your life. We couldn't agree more. There's a better way to do it.

KEEPING TRACK OF FAT INTAKE

The better way comes down to knowing how much fat you're eating daily. Medical authorities urge you to eat no more than 30 percent of your calories as fat. Such advice comes from nutritionists, dietitians, medical establishments, and government organizations, who point out that the percent of fat in the American diet reaches as high as 40 to 45 percent. But what does all this mean in terms of daily living? How can you go into a restaurant or supermarket and order 30 percent fat? Even when we want to follow this health recommendation, doing it is far from easy, and we soon give up.

Now we're going to tell you a simple way to determine and control your fat intake at 30 percent. As we explain this formula, you will understand even more clearly why exercise is essential for good health and desired weight. Remember that lean body mass, or muscle tissue, is your body's engine, and only such tissue burns energy in the form of calories. As you continue your exercise program, you'll develop more lean body mass to burn calories efficiently.

For a sedentary man it takes only about 12 calories to maintain a pound of body weight. If he increases his physical activity to the levels we've been recommending throughout this book, he'll boost the caloric requirement significantly. He will then need 15 calories to maintain a pound of weight. A woman's body, even at ideal weight, contains a higher percentage of fat, and females require fewer calories to maintain weight. For the sedentary woman 9 to 10 calories will maintain a pound of weight; the active woman will burn 13 or 14 calories a pound. The lower the amount of body fat and the higher the amount of lean muscle tissue, the greater the number of calories burned. And the more extensive the exercise program, the more calories burned.

That troublesome word *calorie* keeps popping up, but soon it can be completely forgotten. For the moment, however, let's use it for some calculation. Take two examples, a man and a woman, and assume that both are moderately to extensively engaged in physical exercise, having completed the weight loss phase of this program.

The male wants to maintain his weight at 150 pounds, and the female wants to maintain her 120 pounds. The man will require 15 calories per pound, the woman 13. Total calories for the day, then, will be 2,250 for the man and 1,560 for the woman.

150 pounds × 15 calories = 2,250 calories per day
120 pounds × 13 calories = 1,560 calories per day

Now, how much fat will our man and woman need for the day? We want them both to have 30 percent of their total calories as fat. So we multiply the total calories by 0.30 to give us 675 calories as fat for the man and 468 calories as fat for the woman.

2,250 total calories × 0.30 = 675 calories as fat
1,560 total calories × 0.30 = 468 calories as fat

But how can these examples determine what constitutes 675 or 468 calories as fat? How can they keep track of fat easily? We know that

1 gram of fat supplies 9 calories. So we can easily calculate how many grams of fat should be eaten daily by dividing the calories consumed daily as fat by 9 (the number of calories per gram). For the man this comes out to 75 grams of fat and for the woman, 52.

If the man has 75 grams of fat daily, he'll eat 675 calories as fat. By simply keeping track of that amount of fat, it's highly unlikely that he can possibly consume more than 2,250 total calories for the day while following a balanced diet of good foods. The same holds true for the woman eating 52 grams of fat.

The next step is to be aware of the fat in your diet. How much is 75 grams or 52 grams of fat? The answer can be found in the supermarket. Pick up a quart of milk or a loaf of bread or a can of pasta sauce and you'll see a listing of the amounts of protein, carbohydrates, and fat. After just a while, you'll get to know how much fat there is in a glass of milk, a slice of bread, or a serving of sauce. And you'll know which brands to buy to get the least fat possible.

There are, of course, foods that don't come with a list of nutrients, such as fresh meats, fish, poultry, and fresh produce. That's why we've listed the fat content, along with other nutrient information, of many foods in the table in the Appendix. Spend some time with that table and familiarize yourself with the foods you normally eat. See what they actually contain in terms of fat, protein, and carbohydrates. You don't have to memorize the list, but just by looking it over a few times, you will begin to have a better sense of just how much fat the foods you eat contain.

Would you gulp down a bubbling potion handed to you by a stranger without asking what's in it? Probably not. So why not question what's in the foods you eat? Just as that bubbling potion might be a deadly poison, some of the foods in the supermarkets contain dangerous amounts of the Number One Poison (simple sugars) and the Number One Killer (fats).

Think about the calories coming from fat. As mentioned, each gram of fat contains at least 9 calories, whereas each gram of protein or carbohydrate contains 4. Throughout the weight loss phase of this program we've stressed the importance of choosing lean cuts of meat, fish, and poultry. Making those food selections means that you cut back on fat. In addition to your weight loss, you can experience a significant decline in cholesterol levels. How's that for a nice bonus?

Of course, one mustn't assume that limiting the amount of fat in the diet allows one to go wild with simple carbohydrates as sugars.

The simple sugars are still the Number One Poison when it comes to weight control. But, fortunately, the goals of avoiding excessive amounts of sugar and avoiding fat are not mutually exclusive.

Look at the foods listed in the table in the Appendix, and you'll see how many of the foods high in simple sugars are also high in fat. Cut back on or completely eliminate cookies, pies, cakes, ice cream, and chocolates, and you remove both fat and sugar from your diet. Overweight men and women didn't eat just hard candies for their treats as simple sugars. They, and many if not most other Americans, have been indulging in a deadly combination of the two worst components of the diet, fats and sugars.

ALCOHOL CONSUMPTION

Whether talking about health or weight loss, alcohol inevitably comes up. During weight loss and through stabilization we recommend eliminating alcoholic beverages. There's no way to get around the calories they contribute to the diet, and when greatly restricting calories there's just no room for them.

But at this point you may not want to live without alcohol altogether. First, let's consider the health aspects of drinking. Certainly there's a significant risk of alcoholism, since one of every nine adults in the United States develops this disease. In alcoholics and hard drinkers the liver pays a heavy price. Most deaths from liver disease, a leading cause of death in the United States, are attributable to alcohol abuse. There's no question that pregnant women should avoid alcohol to eliminate fetal alcohol syndrome. And some patients must not drink because of medical conditions such as hepatitis.

On the other hand, moderate alcohol consumption has been widely accepted in this and many other countries and cultures. There are even statistics indicating that moderate drinking is associated with greater longevity. As a specific example, levels of the protective HDL form of cholesterol are higher in drinkers than in nondrinkers, thereby affording some degree of protection from heart disease. The operational term here is "moderate" drinking.

But can one consume alcohol and maintain desired weight? Obviously, the answer is yes, since millions of people do so successfully. But alcoholic beverages are high in calories, and they are "empty" calories, offering no nutritive benefits. Alcohol tends to behave calorically more like a fat than a carbohydrate. It contains about 7 calories per gram, thus somewhere between fat and carbohydrates. (The caloric content of alcoholic beverages is listed in the table in the Appendix.)

Moderate drinking is commonly defined as having no more than a drink or two daily. That might mean a cocktail before dinner or a glass or two of beer or wine with dinner. More than that can put on the pounds not only by way of the added calories but also by lowering your guard against snack foods, which are frequently available at times when significant drinking might occur. What begins as having just a peanut or two winds up as devouring the entire bowlful. It's no coincidence that salty peanuts and pretzels are supplied to tavern patrons; the salt produces thirst, which is quenched by more drinking, followed by more snacking, and on the cycle goes.

We'd also like to throw cold water on the idea of the alcoholic nightcap. There's no worse thing you can do to destroy a good night's sleep. Alcohol before bed is likely to result in a restless night, interruption of deep sleep patterns, and an increased likelihood of awakening in the middle of the night unable to return to sleep. The same applies to the use of alcohol to anesthetize oneself against the adversities of life in general. Instead of that drink, take a brisk walk and a hot bath and read a good book to soothe the nerves; sleep will restore the production of calming serotonin.

Determining just how much you can drink on a regular basis comes down to your personal metabolism. The woman who has a desired weight of only 100 pounds and who does little if any exercise will have a difficult time having even one drink without weight gain. The man who works out regularly in a gym, runs a few miles daily, and weighs 180 pounds of mostly lean tissue will be able to have a martini every night before dinner without gaining an ounce.

View the addition of alcohol to the diet in the same way you approached protein and carbohydrates during the period of stabilization. Have a drink or two in the evening for the next couple of days and check the results on your scale. If you gain weight by adding those alcohol calories while keeping your food calories constant, you'll have to cut down. Perhaps you'll find that one drink daily is your limit. Or maybe you'll prefer having two drinks every other day. As with other foods, you will have to titrate the amount you can ingest without weight gain. The 100-pound woman who finds that she gains weight by having just one drink may decide to make up for the additional calories by increasing her physical activity.

In no case, however, should you substitute alcohol for other foods. Alcohol provides absolutely no nutrition and cannot and should not be exchanged for food. The advice for the 100-pound woman holds true for anyone who finds that desired amounts of alcohol are not compatible with desired weight—get more exercise to burn those excess calories.

LOSING SOME GAINED POUNDS

Remember your first attempts at riding a bicycle? As much as you persevered, you still fell off a lot. Try as you might to listen to all the good advice, you fell. But what happened after the fall? You got right back on and tried again. Finally, you mastered it and wondered how it could ever have been difficult.

As much as we hope that you won't fall when it comes to maintaining your weight, there is a chance it will happen. We're not referring to the 1 or 2 pounds that appear on the bathroom scale after a splurge weekend or a special dinner. You can handle such small deviations from your desired weight simply by cutting back on your carbohydrates and alcohol until the weight returns to normal. By diligently weighing yourself every other day you won't typically gain more than 1 or 2 pounds, and those are rather easily shed now that you know just how your body works in relation to food and exercise.

Those episodes of 1- or 2-pound weight gains are merely slips, not falls. Outright falls are those times when you've completely abandoned your commitment to maintaining your weight.

Today you might shake your head and say, "Never! It won't happen to me. I worked too hard to get that weight off and I'm never going to gain it back!" We hope you're right. And there's no reason to believe that you aren't. Many people have maintained their weight losses for years.

But weight gain can occur. It may follow a major disruption such as a divorce, the loss of a job, or a significant disappointment. Such stresses deplete brain serotonin, which in turn produces strong carbohydrate cravings.

The reasons are not as important as the resultant weight gain. And that weight gain isn't as important as the resolve you must make as quickly as possible to get that weight off again. You've fallen, and now it's time to get right back up on your feet.

Weight regain can be divided into two basic categories: (1) gaining back all or a significant portion of your weight loss and (2) gaining back 5 to 10 pounds, more than can be easily handled by cutting back on a few foods or increasing your daily exercise. In both cases you've slipped back into insulin resistance and the metabolic trap, and you have to get your endocrine system back in order.

As you gain back weight, the same old syndrome returns: depression, water and sodium retention, poor sleep patterns, and an inability to lose the weight by cutting back on calories (even when the fat content of the diet is down to the grams of fat appropriate for your desired weight). The longer you remain in this state of insulin resistance, the more difficult it will be to reverse the process, to return your body to endocrine balance. So, the faster you return to your original commitment the better.

The solution, whether you fall into category 1 or 2, is to reenter the state of ketosis by severely restricting carbohydrates to less than 40 grams. Don't think that just because you've done it once before that you know all there is to know and that you can just call back the program from memory. Start at the beginning. Reread *all* the chapters and begin the program as though you had never done it before. Every chapter has a lesson in it for you. It's time to get back into a regular program of active exercise. It's necessary to relearn your lessons as to the amounts of foods you can eat daily, greatly restricting your carbohydrate intake.

If you've caught yourself when you have gained only 10 or 15 pounds, rather than after you've regained all your lost weight, you'll still have to follow the program as though you need to lose 100 pounds. And regardless of the weight you are now committed to lose, you can count on the program to bring you back to goal weight faster and more efficiently than any other approach.

Once again, start a diet diary, carefully reporting everything you eat and drink during the day and the amount of exercise you do. Note the weight you set as your goal and the daily changes as you get closer to that desired weight.

Do not take any shortcuts. This is the fastest way possible to lose weight safely. Any shortcuts, such as omitting the diary or not doing relaxation techniques (such as deep breathing, meditation, watering flowers, and so forth), will short-circuit the plan.

Take out your diary from the first time you lost weight and compare notes. You'll gain support from reading the progress you made last time and be reliving both the difficult times and the moments of success you recorded at the time.

But most important, you must come to grips with whatever it was that led you away from your commitment to yourself. What has happened to cause you to fall out of love with yourself to such an extent that you have allowed weight gain to occur?

Weight gain of significant proportions isn't simply a matter of having a piece of birthday cake or enjoying a party with all its temptations. You didn't gain that weight because the taste of the food was so wonderful that you just couldn't stop yourself. You know very well that no food in the world can compare to the happiness you feel when you're at your desired weight and feeling terrific.

So get right back to Chapter 6. Read it and reread it. Stand in front of the mirror and say that you love yourself despite what you've done to your body. You're the same person who deserved to lose the weight in the first place, and you deserve to get rid of those extra pounds right now.

Try to view the situation from outside yourself. Would you withhold your fullest love and attention from the dearest person in your life until problems passed? Would you tell your child that you could not love him or her, couldn't do anything for him or her until the conditions changed? Of course not. So why deny that love to the person you should love the most in the whole world—you?

If this is a time of a major disturbance in lifestyle, you might seek professional assistance. It's never a sign of weakness to ask for help. And such support may mean a far easier time in terms of weight loss and getting over your current hurdles.

Tell yourself that you forgive yourself. Give yourself a special treat—a massage, a manicure, or a pedicure—just to show yourself how much you care. You're worth it. And you're worth the effort to get back on track with this program. You did it once, and you can do it again.

We have one word of warning, however. You must be aware that it may be more difficult the

Do not—repeat—do not wait for the emotional or financial turmoil that caused your regain to pass before going back to weight loss and maintenance.

second and subsequent times to get back into ketosis. It's as though you've used this trick on the dragon that guards the metabolic trap before, and now he's wise to your craftiness. That doesn't mean that it's impossible to reenter ketosis, but only that it'll be a bit more difficult. By knowing that in advance, you should be able to cope with the frustration you may feel.

Keep at it. Pretty soon you'll look at yourself in the mirror and congratulate yourself on your weight loss! Now's the time to commit again to maintaining that weight loss permanently. As is true for the person who quits smoking, stops drinking, or quits drugs, it's not the times you tried and slipped or fell that count, it's the time you finally succeeded permanently. The former smoker and the recovering alcoholic do not think about anything except his or her current freedom from addiction. Now that you're at your desired weight, enjoy your success and your good health. You've done it and you're glad.

Congratulations!

Increased serotonin from nighttime trazodone can be remarkably effective. The secret of successful and permanent weight loss is insulin control—by diet and exercise—and serotonin enhancement from good sleep aided by trazodone, under the direction of your doctor.

▪ ▪ ▪

As you read these pages you may feel that this is all very complicated and you'll have a difficult time keeping track of all the elements—fat, carbohydrates, protein, alcohol, and exercise—in order to permanently maintain your goal weight For you, as for anyone embarking on a new venture, we can only offer the encouragement that it will soon become second nature to you. Think of the time when you first learned to ride a bicycle, ski down a hill, or hit a golf ball straight down the fairway. Your instructor told you to do several things at once and you thought at the time that it was impossible to do so. But you persevered, learned, and succeeded. You will succeed at weight maintenance as well.

Chapter 10

LIFE CHANGES AND SUPPORT STRATEGIES FOR SUCCESS

Whether you have always been heavy or put on weight later in life, food played only a partial role in your overweight development. Those who believe that simply sticking to a diet will make unwanted pounds disappear permanently are due for certain failure. The only way to achieve lasting success is to restructure your lifestyle in a meaningful way. As effective as the Insulin Control Diet is, the program is incomplete and harder to follow without some lifestyle changes. The methods described in this chapter will help reduce stress and strengthen compliance.

You might be convinced that it's food, not lifestyle or behavior, that's been your problem. If you have just 2 or 3 pounds to lose, you are probably right. Even weight gains of 5 to 10 pounds, say after a long vacation or over the holidays, can frequently be coped with if one has sufficient motivation. But as much as we wish it weren't so, one scientific fact remains: excessive weight is a long-term result of too much insulin and too little serotonin, leading to too many calories and too little exercise. Often as a person gains weight because of poor sleep and uncontrolled carbohydrate cravings he or she does even less physical activity. And, if those pounds remain as fat tissue and you continue to gain weight, the problems of the endocrine system kick in. Wrong foods eaten at the wrong times for the wrong reasons make the metabolic trap close even tighter. So foods and the diet must be viewed as part of the total lifestyle.

A MATTER OF MOTIVATION

Most decisions in life seem relatively unimportant. We can decide to start playing golf and later decide to give it up and sell the clubs. We can change hairstyles, and if we don't like them, the hair will grow back. But there are some decisions that require a concerted commitment backed by heartfelt motivation.

How do you develop the motivation to make weight control a sustained effort? With diabetes and those with a family history of the disease, it is entirely an intellectual decision. Live longer with relatively good health or die prematurely from the ravages of diabetes, which include heart disease, blindness, kidney failure, gangrene, and neuropathy. However, to achieve and maintain success in weight loss requires a degree of passion. Think about it. Don't you have enough passion in your life to save your own life?

LOVING YOURSELF AND EXPECTED LIFE CHANGES

Certainly one needs to modify behavior for long-term success, and many of the behavior modification tricks and techniques we read about in magazines are useful. But more fundamentally, and as a first step to revamping your lifestyle, you probably need to change your attitude.

Your approach to living comes down first to loving. Do you really love yourself? Enough to want the very best for yourself? Enough to do whatever it takes to get the very best?

If you answered yes to loving yourself, how can it be that you've been willing to carry the extra pounds that prevent the fullest enjoyment of life and threaten life itself? If you answered no, perhaps you are not giving yourself enough credit for loving. You did, after all, start reading this book, didn't you? Probably you do love yourself and have the potential to do so, but just as we don't always act in loving ways to those who are dear to us, we don't always know *how* to love ourselves faithfully and fully. It can be difficult to love yourself when the world seems to condemn you for being overweight. Even parents, if they're not overweight themselves, criticize children for those extra pounds. And every glance in the mirror seems to confirm the world's opinions: How can I love myself when I look like this?

It's time to make a commitment to loving yourself unconditionally. We're not so naive as to believe you can simply make that deci-

> Once a person has become substantially insulin resistant, weight loss becomes difficult if not impossible, especially on a permanent basis.

sion and have it happen like some sort of lightning bolt out of the sky. It may have taken quite a few years to fall out of love with yourself, and it may take a while to fall back in love. There was a time when you did love yourself completely and unconditionally. As children, we all had innate self-love. We had to learn not to love ourselves. And now it's time to regain that childlike self-love.

Just as a marriage counselor might advise a squabbling couple to reacquaint themselves, remembering the things that first drew them together as a couple, we advise you to give yourself a chance to learn what a terrific person you really are. You're not just OK. You're wonderful!

Take a moment right now to jot down a few particularly nice things about yourself. Perhaps you are honest, trustworthy, or devoted to duty. Maybe you are especially willing to give of yourself to others. You might have career and professional achievements. Think about the physical features you've gotten compliments about through the years—your hair, your eyes, your skin. Almost every person has at least one or two beautiful features. Have you forgotten about yours?

Even if you find it easier to think of your flaws, why not view your flawed self with the same compassion you give to the other people you love? Do you expect them to be perfect? Do you withhold love from them when they're not? You really are worth loving. You don't have to earn love by being perfect. To love yourself on an unconditional basis means doing so today, not waiting until you lose those pounds. Not waiting until you get your promotion, but today. Not when you find someone who tells you they love you, but today. There's no reason to be reserved or cautious; love yourself absolutely.

Next, prove your love for yourself by doing some nice things for yourself. Go to the bookstore and buy that book you've been wanting to read. Go to a movie. Bring home fresh flowers from the supermarket. Make it a point to do something particularly nice for yourself every week. And every day give yourself at least a gesture of your own esteem. Every person loves to hear someone say, "I love you." Start saying that to yourself daily, not only in words but in deeds. Look yourself in the mirror and say, "I really do love you." As someone who is truly loved, you want the best for yourself.

No turning back or finding excuses this time. You know you're in good medical hands, and this is the best possible program. After all, you don't want someone you love to be at increased risk of disease, do you? Reducing weight will reduce that risk. You want someone you love to live a long time, and this program can increase longevity. And you want your loved ones to feel good about themselves and be full of energy.

How can you ensure that commitment to the program? You need more than willpower; you need assistance in developing self-control. You could check into a clinic and have your environment and your diet controlled for you. You definitely would lose weight, but if you didn't learn techniques for making this a permanent lifestyle change, it's very likely that you would gain the weight back.

You've already taken the first step in changing your lifestyle by making the commitment to love yourself. And you've placed your faith in the ability of this program to help you lose weight. There are also behavioral changes you can make that will enhance your success. But it's not just a matter of learning techniques; rather, you must make a commitment to doing those things that can help remove the harmful habits that have contributed to your overweight condition. We're not just talking about tricks, such as using smaller plates to make food appear more plentiful. We're referring to new ways of dealing with your environment and the food in that environment. You can't possibly change all the negative behaviors in your life in a day, a week, or even a month. Give yourself the time it takes to make some real and profound changes. Read this chapter over and over again until the message really sinks in.

Take a few minutes to review your own reasons for wanting to lose weight at this moment in life. These can be vital sources of inspiration when the program seems difficult. One good way to focus on your personal motivation for achieving and maintaining your goal weight is to think about the ways your life will change when you succeed.

Make a list of how your life will change, or if you're at your goal weight, how it has changed already. Write down your feelings, and then come back to review your words from time to time.

Part of giving yourself the best is making an absolute commitment to this program.

You'll find that by doing so you'll strengthen your resolve, both by reminding yourself of your reasons and by the satisfaction of seeing the predicted changes coming true.

The changes you can expect will be in a number of areas, some more important to you than others. We've provided a few guidelines, but feel free to add others, or write your own list.

- Life Changes Expected in Personal Growth
- Life Changes Expected in Self-Esteem
- Life Changes Expected in Health
- Life Changes Expected in Career
- Life Changes Expected in Social Life

CLARIFYING GOALS

The expectations of change are your motivation to realize your weight loss goals. Now let's look at what those goals are. Set realistic goals. You may not expect to become a fashion model (unless you were one before gaining weight), but you do have distinct goals. Nearly all successful people do set definite and achievable goals in order to turn dreams into reality. By seeing the light at the end of the tunnel, you can focus your efforts more clearly, and you can start to measure your success on a step-by-step basis.

Let's turn to the analogy of a college education. That is the goal for a freshman first setting foot on campus. But to get to that goal, he or she must first achieve some significant subgoals, such as completing a course, passing an examination, writing a thesis, and so forth. Looking at the pile of books, reports, and tests a student must get through in the coming years would be enough to make any freshman turn tail and run. Instead, the freshman will pick up the books and assignments for that first semester and go on from there. Sticking with it, our freshman will become a sophomore, then a junior, and finally a senior. Graduation day arrives. As the saying goes, inch by inch it's a cinch, but yard by yard it's very hard.

What are your broad goals? How many pounds do you want to lose? Focus on a realistic, achievable goal. Perhaps that goal is the weight you remember in high school or before your baby was born or before your career started gobbling all your time.

And there's more to this program than just lost pounds. You will also achieve a gradual but certain reduction in your measurements. In fact, even at times when it seems as though the pounds aren't disappearing as you hoped they would, the inches will continue to decrease.

Before starting the program, take a few minutes to measure your body. Write the measurements down, both pounds and inches, on the Body Measurement Record (Table 10.1). Mark the date. Then return to note your improvements over time.

Now it's time to start clarifying your picture of your soon-to-be self. Close your eyes and imagine yourself with those pounds and inches reduced. Bring that picture into sharper focus by mentally arranging your clothing. Are you wearing a suit, slacks and sweater, or swimsuit? Are you standing in your office or on the beach? Is the picture the way you appeared a few years ago?

If you were once the weight you now want to achieve, you can help clarify your mental image by looking at a photograph taken when you were at your desired weight. If no such photos are available, scan through a few magazines until you find a picture of someone you can model yourself after. But be realistic. Looking at pictures in *Playboy, Vogue,* or *GQ* won't do the trick. Concentrate on that picture of yourself. Burn it into your consciousness as one of the major accomplishments for the future and one of the most important efforts today. In the coming weeks you'll want to call that image up every day in your mind, and each week you'll be closer to looking like that mental image.

As a sign of commitment to attaining and maintaining his or her goal weight, a formerly overweight person should simply get rid of oversized clothes. Keeping large clothes in the closet is inviting the inevitable weight gain. By keeping them, you're actually saying that your ideal weight is only temporary, and you'll be ready for the return of your old weight. Jackie Gleason kept three full wardrobes at all times, in large, medium, and slender sizes. He had no real expectation at any time to keep his weight down.

Some of the people who have succeeded most dramatically in losing weight have had their clothes taken in by a tailor every step of the way. Those who can afford to do so buy new outfits to keep up

Table 10.1 Body Measurement Record

Date	Pounds	Waist	Hips	Upper Thighs	Arms	Chest

with their changing figures. None keep the old sizes hanging in the closet.

You've made a commitment to weight loss, and this time you really mean it. If you had just enrolled in college, you'd tell your friends and relatives. So tell them now that you've decided that with the help of this book and its program you're going to lose the weight that has been adversely affecting your life. Tell them in strong, positive tones.

You're accomplishing a great deal by such a declaration to everyone around you. By telling them now that you no longer will eat certain foods, they won't be surprised later. You won't be tempted to have that special something your mother or friend cooked or baked "just for you." If they persist in their temptations, remind them that you informed them clearly and unequivocally that you wouldn't be eating that food until your goal has been reached.

You'll also be burning bridges behind you. There's no turning back on your commitment. You've told these people that you'll be losing weight on a regular and predictable basis. So now you'll have to deliver on your promise. But remember that it's *you*, not them, to whom your promise really matters.

When you make your announcements, enlist the help and support of all those around you. We all need all the help we can get, especially when it comes to particularly important projects. And when it comes to weight loss, friends and relatives can actually sabotage your efforts more effectively than all the television and magazine food ads you can imagine. We'll give you some specific defenses against such sabotage later in this chapter. But people like to be asked for help, and when they think their contributions will be of value, they are often eager to cooperate.

Would one or more of your friends like to lose weight also? Perhaps you can establish a little circle of support by doing the program together. Having a friend or two to lose weight with can help you get through some of the tougher moments of temptation and frustration. Some of the greater successes with this program have been with patients who followed the program together.

But beware of the flip side to this coin. If your friend does not make a complete commitment to the program in the same way that you have, he or she could become a barrier to your success. Having abandoned the diet in favor of a box of chocolates and a cheesecake, your friend may well attempt to get you off the program as well. He or she can make it more difficult for you, and the last thing you need is sabotage.

PHYSICAL ACTIVITY

What you do need, however, is physical activity. We discussed exercise in Chapter 7, but here we are talking about physical activity as a part of one's lifestyle. It's a matter of movement. Some overweight people have made an art of avoiding all but the most necessary physical movements. They cruise around trying to find parking places directly in front of stores, rather than park a block away and walk there. They take elevators and escalators, rather than climb stairs. They order merchandise from catalogs, rather than go to a store to shop. They even use prepared foods, rather than cook from scratch.

The result of such lack of movement is that the calorie-burning engine shuts down. With so little muscular activity, the body stores rather than uses incoming fuels. The person consumes more calories than necessary to provide for energy needs, increasing stored fat with its insulin-resistant properties. In this way you develop an inevitable progressive state of obesity.

In addition to your daily exercise program, increase the amount of movement in your everyday life. But don't do it just because we're telling you to; do it because you love yourself. The next time you have a chance to climb stairs, do so. When you go shopping or out to an appointment, park the car at least a block away from the door. As time goes on, make that a block and a half and then two blocks.

Modern technology has given us a number of convenient work savers. Start turning them off. Use the old-fashioned way of getting things done. Chop vegetables by hand instead of using the food processor when making family meals. Every little bit helps to burn calories and increase your body's metabolic rate. When secretaries were given electric typewriters to replace their manual machines in a study done many years ago, the women uniformly gained weight. You'd never imagine that such a little thing would matter. But, again, every little bit helps or hurts.

RELAXING ACTIVITIES

While we want you to do more physical activity, we also want you to relax more and to do so more often. That's not really a contradiction. A relaxed person will sleep better and will awaken refreshed to start another day of physical activity. But just as overweight people have often forgotten how to exercise, they also have lost track of beneficial relaxation.

The person who has made lack of movement an art form might think not doing anything is a kind of relaxation. But sitting and watching television with the aid of the remote control does not necessarily promote a relaxed, peaceful state; often quite the opposite is true, since activity loosens (relaxes) muscles.

At the opposite extreme is the person who works continually and "has no time" to relax. But there's always time to grab a calorie-laden snack, or to become upset over a traffic snarl, or to have three martinis before dinner to calm down.

A relaxed person is less likely to reach for food.

Both extremes need to take the time to learn some techniques to make their periods of relaxation more productive in terms of losing weight and enjoying life in general. Once again, the first step is to make a commitment to doing some relaxing activities every day. We use the term "relaxing activities" to emphasize that what we're recommending is more than doing nothing. You have to put some concentrated energy into being fully relaxed.

As with exercise, a type of relaxing activity that works well for one person might not be effective for another. Some relaxation techniques can be done alone, while others involve a group. And some types require some equipment. Finding something that works for you and that you can and will do regularly is the key to success.

At the beginning many people find that they appreciate assistance. For them a yoga or meditation class can be helpful. Today such classes are offered in practically every community. Check out the programs at the local YMCA as well as those offered in health clubs, spas, and gyms.

Yoga is a system of physical poses and postures that enables one to concentrate on relaxing both mind and body. It brings one more in tune with one's body, especially after perhaps years of inactivity, and it helps limber up unused joints. Once the techniques are learned, yoga exercises can be done at home, at the office, or on vacation. And one can continue to attend classes for group support.

Meditation classes teach techniques for concentrating more fully on bringing the mind and body to a state of relaxed awareness. One type of meditation, biofeedback, uses an apparatus designed to measure galvanic skin response (in the same way lie detectors work) to determine the state of anxiety or relaxation an individual is in. Using this principle on a crude level, one could hold a fever thermometer in the grip of one's hand and read the temperature. A cold reading indicates stress, while a warm reading, in the range of the mid-80s, denotes relaxation. By then concentrating purposefully on raising the skin temperature, the state of relaxation deepens. Biofeedback devices are available to help that concentration by providing a constant tone on which to focus one's ideas, thus ridding the mind of irritating thoughts.

Most of us are unable to go for long without falling victim to negative thoughts and feelings. But as time goes on, especially with the assistance of relaxation techniques, we can improve our ability to concentrate on a pleasant concept or a neutral tone in order to relax.

If you prefer to begin your efforts in relaxation on your own, a few suggestions can help you succeed. Select a location where you can be alone for ten to fifteen minutes at a time. That may mean disconnecting the telephone for a while, telling your secretary to hold calls, or not responding to e-mails. It may necessitate going off to a separate room, into the garage, or sitting in a parked car.

Darken the area as much as possible. You may find that some types of music can help you stop thinking about everyday problems. The so-called New Age music is specifically designed to do just that. Such music is restful, employing soft guitar strains, harpstylings, and electronically engineered sound effects. Try listening to a recording with headphones. Then close your eyes and conjure up a pleasant idea or memory. This is called *imagery*.

Such imagery has been proven amazingly effective and beneficial in blocking out much of the world around you. In some cases an individual—a teacher, group leader, therapist, or even friend—will guide the imagery by telling a subject to concentrate on a given scene, describing that scene as it evolves. Perhaps it will be a guided mental tour through a path in the woods or a stroll down a beach.

Details of the landscape, the scattered pinecones or the driftwood washed to shore, are brought to mind, as the listener focuses thoughts entirely on that scene.

This guided imagery has been used by cancer specialists to help patients receiving chemotherapy. By concentrating on a soothing, peaceful scene, the patient can block out the negative images of the medication being injected. Frequently the nausea often associated with chemotherapy can be eliminated by using guided imagery.

Give imagery a try when you begin to take moments out from your day to relax. You'll find that your skills will grow with practice. In time you'll be able to transport yourself to the scene of your choice—a beach, park, forest, or desert. Describe to yourself all the elements of your picture, as though you were describing it to a blind person.

In fact, you can go further and guide yourself in imagery relating to your weight. Draw a mental picture of yourself as you would like to appear. Daily refer to that mental image and compare it with your current weight, noting how the pounds and inches are disappearing. Many patients have found such imagery to be astoundingly effective and have succeeded at weight loss far better than others who do not use this technique.

As with exercise, your relaxation practices should not be limited to a specified period of time daily. Try to find frequent, short periods of time when you can relax. If you're caught in a traffic jam during rush hour, focus on pleasant thoughts, put on some relaxing music, and concentrate on not becoming irritated by the delays. If you are waiting for a late appointment, don't fret and keep looking at your watch. Instead, take the time to close your eyes and relax. Or take along some light reading so you can pass the time enjoyably.

Working the art of relaxation by meditation into your daily routine can assist your weight loss efforts.

MODIFYING YOUR FOOD BEHAVIOR

A key to permanent weight loss is to broaden the scope of your lifestyle horizons to avoid situations that have contributed to your weight gain. By that we mean replacing food-related situations with those that are incompatible with eating. Instead of continually munching on snacks while watching television, engage in an activity using your hands. It's hard to grab for a potato chip when you're knitting or building a ship in a bottle. Not only do such hobbies eliminate the temptation to snack, but they also help you relax. Instead of centering social engagements around food, make other plans with friends, such as a walk at the botanical gardens or a drive to the beach.

The only way to zero in on all your food habits is to keep a strict food diary. Record everything you put into your mouth, both food and beverages, including when you take a drink to wash down medications or vitamins. Note the time of day, where you are when you consume, and the circumstances. You

Record your victories in your diet diary.

might comment, for example, that you ate or drank something because you received bad news or because you needed a reward for getting through a tough time. Be sure to make daily entries and keep the diary not just for a day or a week but for the months while you lose weight and learn to keep the pounds and inches off permanently.

Next, do some planning. If you have a party to go to, you know that food and drink will be served and that friends and relatives will urge you to have "just a little." Plan for that in advance. What are you going to say? How will you keep your hands busy? When offered a drink, there's no need to order a glass of water with a dour expression on your face. Instead, ask for a Perrier on ice with a twist of lemon peel. The attitude you take and the appearance of the drink can make all the difference in the world.

Read back through your diary now and then to see how much easier it's becoming to stick to the program. Entries at the beginning may reflect difficulties that are no longer problems a few weeks later.

We'd like to share with you some ways to modify your behavior when it comes to food. Make an effort to implement these techniques and make them a regular part of your lifestyle.

Many good intentions for proper dieting are abandoned in the aisles of the supermarket. There are some definite dos and don'ts that can eliminate the hazards of shopping. Practice them regularly and they'll become an automatic part of your behavior.

Plan your grocery shopping on a weekly basis and do not vary from your shopping list, even if you see a spectacular buy. Prepare that list after, not before, a meal. The same applies to the shopping itself. Never go to the store on an empty stomach. Plan menus for a week, and put on your shopping lists all the ingredients you need for the meals. Such planning will not only help you to stay on the diet but will make life easier by making it organized.

If you are planning meals for others besides yourself, whenever possible, try to center the meal around the foods that you'll be eating as part of the diet. The others can simply have more of those foods than you will. Perhaps a side dish or two can fill out their calorie needs. Remember, too, that *everyone* will be better off cutting back on fat.

Don't shop from memory. If you've forgotten your list, go home and get it. Don't shop with others, unless they are also on the diet. Don't tempt yourself by buying snack foods or foods that were your favorites. And don't buy more food than you'll need for that week.

When you come home from shopping, immediately put all foods away out of sight. If you must keep snack foods in the house for other members of the family, keep those foods far away from areas you use frequently. If possible, have the children keep such foods in their rooms in tightly closed containers. Perhaps your spouse can take such foods to the office or other workplace. Explain to your family that, at least for a while, just seeing those foods can sway you from your good intentions. Keeping them stored away will be an act of love on your family's part. It's a small thing to ask.

If there are foods in the house that you were particularly fond of and other members of the family don't eat, it's best to throw them out if you can't give them away. Don't worry about the waste.

Make it difficult for yourself to get to food quickly. Store foods in nontransparent containers so you can't see them. Remove the light bulb in the refrigerator to make it more difficult to find foods. Discard any leftovers lest you become tempted to eat them just to get them out of the house. Perhaps you can feed leftovers to your dog so you're not wasting food.

If you prepare food for your family, whenever possible do it after you have already eaten. Cooking on an empty stomach can test the strongest resolve. Other family members can also eat the foods you'll be eating on this diet as well as carbohydrate items that you'll avoid. Everyone can benefit by reducing fat intake. Again, ask them to go along with this out of love for you. But if it can't be done, don't let their foods tempt you.

While you're cooking, food aromas can be stimulating to the point of distraction. Minimize those aromas by turning on the kitchen exhaust fan and by covering pots of simmering foods.

Especially at the start of the program, stick entirely with the recipes provided in this book. Measure ingredients accurately to be sure you're not consuming calories and carbohydrates you're not aware of.

This is the time to learn to measure food properly. To do so, you'll need some basic kitchen equipment. Buy a good food scale that weighs foods down to a fraction of an ounce. If you don't already have them, get measuring cups and spoons. Don't rely on your perceived notion of what an ingredient weighs or measures in volume. Take the time to make measuring a routine part of cooking. It'll help now and in the many years to come.

The recipes call for specific amounts of ingredients, all designed to stay within daily calorie limits and to maintain ketosis by restricting carbohydrates. Needless to say, it will defeat the purpose of such recipes if the ingredients are not measured precisely. During the period of stabilization and maintenance, when you are gradually adding portions of foods, you'll also want those portions to be properly measured to ensure success.

When serving foods, put only the proper amounts on the table. Don't tempt yourself into taking second helpings. If your family eats with you, put your food on your own plate in the kitchen and don't eat from any other plates or serving utensils.

We start changing eating behavior by assessing when and where food will be eaten. Many overweight individuals eat on an almost continuous basis throughout the day. A careful and honest review of your routine will put your eating habits into perspective for you. As part of this program, we ask you to restrict your eating to three meals and two snacks per day. That's five eating times daily, and that should be enough to satisfy. If you've been eating more frequently than that, you'll have to break that habit to end the years of overweight.

Not only do we want you to limit yourself to three meals and two snacks each day, but we want you to eat those three meals and two snacks every day. Don't try to improve on the diet or to speed up your progress by skipping meals. We want you not only to lose weight, but also to learn proper eating habits for the rest of your life. That means scheduling regular meals. We emphasize the word *regu-*

lar because it's best to have those meals at just about the same times each day. Many overweight individuals got that way by skipping a meal here and there and "making up for it" with huge meals later on in the day. Eating regular meals will help stabilize your blood sugar and insulin level.

Remember, too, *why* you must eat. Although we all enjoy the tastes, appearances, and aromas of foods; the pleasures of physically chewing and swallowing; and the social rituals of eating, the basic reason we eat is to give our bodies nourishment. We should eat to live, rather than live to eat. All other reasons must be considered secondary, especially the many reasons we use to justify our unnecessary eating. We snack at parties to be social and celebrate. We gorge when feeling sorry for ourselves. We nibble to keep ourselves company when we're alone. We munch to have something to do with our hands while doing something entirely unrelated.

We've discussed why we eat and when; yet *where* we eat can be equally important. Especially if you've been eating virtually nonstop from morning till night, or if you've concentrated your eating into a period of the day, such as in the evening starting with dinner and ending with bedtime, you've been eating everywhere. Food has accompanied you into the living room, bedroom, laundry room, bathroom, office, car, and beyond. Beginning now, there's only one proper place to eat your meals—the dining-room table.

For many overweight patients that's a stiff order, one that takes a lot of getting used to. But simply limiting your food consumption to the dinner table will automatically eliminate a large portion of calories typically consumed. It also allows you to concentrate on eating, which will make you more satisfied.

At designated times of the day, prepare your food and serve it to yourself at the table, even if the table is outside the home, at the office, or elsewhere. Make the plate of food attractive, perhaps by garnishing with parsley or a sprig of mint. Look forward to eating the food and enjoy every bite. Eat it without gulping. We want to slow down the process of eating.

Some well-known techniques of behavior modification for weight loss involve slowing down the speed of food consumption. The researchers who first suggested this approach made the assumption that overweight men and women eat their food rapidly and that by slowing the process down they would eat less food and be more satisfied by it. While there is no evidence that overweight individuals eat any faster than slender people, by following some of these suggestions, one can decrease the amount of food consumed and enhance enjoyment of it. Even if you feel that you don't currently wolf down meals, you will benefit by employing some of the following suggestions.

Take small bites of food. Concentrate on tasting the food rather than swallowing it immediately. Focus on the effect of the food on your lips, teeth, and tongue. Chew it thoroughly. Decades ago, a researcher named Horace Fletcher advocated the chewing of each mouthful of food exactly twenty-eight times. The nation was filled with people "Fletcherizing" their food. While his rationale for the practice—it aids proper digestion—has fallen under criticism and the practice is no longer followed, chewing food thoroughly has other benefits.

Swallow *before* you take the next bite. Put down your knife and fork while chewing, thus making a distinct separation between mouthfuls of food. You can practice becoming a food dallier by deliberately taking breaks in eating a meal. Even after food has been swallowed, wait a few seconds before cutting off the next bite. As time goes on, those delays between mouthfuls can increase from those few seconds up to half a minute and more.

Regardless of the type of food you're eating, use utensils. Even if nibbling at finger foods, use a fork, if possible, to pick up the morsels. This helps to make you pay attention to what and how much you are eating, rather than absentmindedly putting food in your mouth. You might even try to eat some meals with chopsticks to slow the process down further.

When you're finished with your food at that meal, don't delay at the table. Get up and immediately clean off the plates, utensils, and cookware. If you're cleaning the plates of others, don't be tempted into taking even the smallest taste of any leftover uneaten food. Remind yourself that you will eat only what is on your plate while you are seated at the dinner table.

In all matters related to food for you and your family, try to enlist the cooperation of others. If they're not already doing so, your children and spouse can certainly share in the chores. In fact, the more you can separate yourself from the family's foods during the initial period of weight loss, the better off you'll be. And you'll also save yourself and your family from the anger and resentment that might arise in you when as a dieting person you must prepare, serve, and clean up after the meals that you're unable to enjoy personally.

SUPPORT STRATEGIES

Love yourself enough to enlist the help of others. Expect them to love you enough to provide that help and to support your weight loss efforts, not sabotage them.

It can be difficult, but you can do it. The suggestions that follow are designed to help you in the coming days, weeks, and months of your weight loss and maintenance. Try reading only one section at a time, and integrate each suggestion into your life before going on to the next. In time, you'll be actively engaged in following several recommendations at once.

Support Strategy 1: Tell the World

You've made a commitment to weight loss; this time you know you'll succeed. It's time to tell your friends, relatives, associates, and anyone who could possibly have an influence on your eating habits the good news. Tell them you've begun a program you have confidence in and that you will not sway from your resolve no matter what.

> Most important, love yourself enough to follow through with your weight loss commitment even if you don't get the support of others.

This is the time to be assertive. You don't have to be nasty in rejecting their offers of foods and drinks. To assert oneself, *Webster's New World Dictionary* states, is to insist on one's rights. Surely you have a right to be healthy and happy, and that's really what weight loss is all about.

If necessary, make a list of everyone who might be in a position to affect your diet. Make it a point to talk with each person before a food situation comes up. Don't wait until you're visiting someone's home and he or she asks you to have "just one slice of this cake—I made it just for you." After all, you're a nice person, and you don't want to hurt anyone's feelings.

Explain to people that you're on "doctor's orders" not to eat certain foods. If further explanation is required, tell them that your body cannot tolerate simple carbohydrates, and for a while you're following a strict dietary regimen that's been medically documented to help those with conditions such as yours. It will be up to you if you want to go into the details of insulin resistance. But, regardless of circumstances, make it clear that you will not accept foods and drinks not permitted in the weight loss program. Perhaps you've never before been forceful about something terribly important to you. This is a good time to start.

One patient described what was, in perspective, an amusing story of how she had to "fight off" offers of a sweet potato pie during the Christmas holidays. Her hostess maintained that the pie was baked with absolutely no sugar. She didn't take into consideration that the pie consisted almost entirely of other carbohydrates. And to make matters even more amusing, she had substituted maple syrup for the sugar, since "that's natural." Moreover, the hostess said, "I baked it just for you." How can someone refuse an offer like that? But the patient did refuse, and she was proud of it.

Like so many things in life, the first time you refuse forbidden foods is the hardest. Sure, you'll be tempted. But if you've told your friends about your program, you won't want to fail in front of them. They'll be watching to see how you do. And as you say no to this and no to that, and tell more and more people that you're on this program, you start to feel real pride.

If you were a recovering alcoholic, it's unlikely your friends and loved ones would offer you a drink. If you had quit smoking cigarettes, they wouldn't constantly tempt you with "just one puff." Your program is just as important. You're doing it because you love yourself. If other people love you, they'll help, not hinder, your efforts.

Support Strategy 2: Keep the Cookie Jar Filled

Do you have a cookie jar that you keep filled with snacks for yourself and your family? Judith did, and she couldn't bring herself to put it away or to leave it empty on the kitchen counter. It was so cozy to have that cookie jar filled, but the temptation was horrid.

So Judith came up with a solution. Instead of cookies, she filled the jar with dog biscuits. That served a number of purposes. Obviously, she wasn't tempted to munch on them. Second, the cookie jar reminded her that she promised herself that she wouldn't give up the diet. And third, visitors to the house got an amusing, dramatic display of Judith's resolve.

If that approach is not quite up your alley, and you have a cookie jar that begs for filling, here's an idea that will help you today and for the rest of your life. Instead of sweet, caloric treats, fill your cookie jar with sweet, nonfood treats. Write ideas and suggestions for treats for yourself on pieces of paper and fill the jar with them. When you dip into the cookie jar, you'll pull out another way to give yourself a lift. Here are a few suggestions to put into the jar:

- Take a long, restful bubble bath.
- Give yourself a pedicure, complete with nail polish if you like.
- Make a phone call to someone you haven't spoken with in a long time. List some friends to call.
- Read a book you've been dying to read.
- Take a nap for just a few minutes to recharge your energies. Set a timer for five or ten minutes.
- Make an appointment to get a massage.
- Write yourself a poem.
- Curl up for fifteen minutes with a magazine.
- Work on a crossword puzzle.
- Do some knitting or crocheting.
- Ask your spouse if he or she wouldn't enjoy a "matinee." It's more fun to reach for a mate instead of a plate!
- Take care of a chore you've been putting off. (This one could probably fill a few slips of paper.) You'll be so glad to have finally done it!
- Pull out a CD and listen to a song you haven't heard for a while.
- For women, fix your hair for the evening; do something fun with it. Perhaps braid in some colorful ribbon.
- Measure your lost inches.
- Take clothes to the tailor for alterations.

Think of things that really appeal to you. You can make those slips of paper more festive by rolling them into scrolls and tying them with ribbon. As you think of new ideas, keep adding them to the cookie jar. Be on the lookout for new ideas in magazines. Enjoy your sweet treats!

Support Strategy 3: Make a Deal

Lawyers use the phrase *quid pro quo*, literally, "this for that." Here's an example of how one patient used the concept of quid pro quo to lose weight.

Dorothy's husband had urged her to shed her extra pounds for quite a while. She, on the other hand, had hoped he would help with some household chores. So she offered a quid pro quo deal. George accepted, thinking that Dorothy wouldn't go through with her commitment. He began to help with the chores, and Dorothy began to follow the program.

To George's surprise, Dorothy stayed with it. When he neglected his share of the chores, she reminded him of the deal. And, when Dorothy started to waver in her resolve, George mentioned how he really didn't want to do those dishes that night. George and Dorothy resolved two difficulties in their marriage with one deal. Both were happy with the outcome.

Maybe this particular quid pro quo wouldn't work for you. Maybe you don't have a spouse to make a deal with. Perhaps you could make a deal with yourself. Is there something you'd really like to do or have? Something you've been denying yourself for quite some time? Perhaps it's a vacation or a trip to visit friends or family. Maybe it's a new piece of furniture or a subscription to a theater series. Most of us have something that we've denied ourselves for too long. So make a deal with yourself. Set a goal weight as the condition for realizing that dream.

Let's say it's the vacation that's part of your quid pro quo. Go to the travel agency and get some brochures and details of the trip. Find out when the flights depart. Mark your calendar for the date you'll leave. Go to the library or bookstore and find some reading material on your destination, and whenever you start to slip or feel tempted, read about your paradise. Let the world know about it. Tell your friends that if you lose those pounds you're on your way.

Another way to arrange a deal with yourself is to promise that if you don't lose the weight, you'll deprive yourself of something you already have. That was the case for hundreds of police officers in Louisiana who were told that if they didn't conform to weight regulations, they would lose their jobs. That was enough negative motivation for all of them to comply and to lose the excess weight. Certainly you won't consider as drastic a deal as was forced upon those police officers. Your self-imposed deprivation must be more realistic in terms of your life, perhaps not going to a movie or concert as planned until you lose a specified amount of weight.

Whether you think you'd do better with positive or negative motivation, make your quid pro quo deal an act of love. Never forget: You're worth loving—you love yourself!

Support Strategy 4: Invest in Weight Loss

"Money talks." "You get what you pay for." "What's it worth to you?" These and other expressions in our language reveal the importance we all, to one degree or another, place on money. So let's see how you might relate weight loss to dollars.

If you were to go to a local weight loss center, you would pay a considerable sum of money for the program it offers. Some are more expensive than others, but even the least expensive programs will cost about $10 for each pound to be lost. Costs at some commercial weight loss operations double or triple that amount. And they typically want their money, or at least most of it, right up front before you shed the first ounce.

What is your current financial status? Could you afford $10, $20, or $30 per pound? Do you have 20, 40, or 100 pounds to lose? You can make the calculation quite easily as to what weight loss in your case would cost. Would it be worth that amount of money? Of course it would. How can one set a price for health and happiness? So here's a strategy that has worked well.

Determine the amount of money you will "pay" to lose those pounds and inches. Take that money and put it into a bank, give it to a friend, or make some other arrangement to keep it stashed away.

Then make a deal to get the money back. Instead of paying others to help you lose weight, pay yourself for getting the job done.

Set up a payment schedule. Draw out a given amount of money for each week you remain in ketosis. Or, predicate the payment on achieving a given amount of weight loss per week. Or, pay yourself for each inch lost or each pound lost or both.

Regardless of the terms of payment, however, you must make the promise that if you fail to deliver on your deal, you don't get paid. Not only that, but the money should be forfeited *forever*. Contribute the lost funds to a charity. Tell a close friend about your financial arrangement to make sure you can't get out of it. The most effective means of enforcing the arrangement is to have the friend be completely responsible for the money. Thus, each week he or she will either send you the amount you have earned or send it to the charity. Complying fully with the program means you lose nothing.

It's possible, of course, that you could lose all the money you set aside, but we don't think you will swell the treasuries of charities by much at all. This program is so effective that if you stick to it you're guaranteed success. Put your money where your mouth is!

Support Strategy 5: Take a Shortcut to Feeling Good

What's the most intensely pleasurable memory you can think of that has nothing to do with food? Perhaps it was staring at the stars in a black sky aboard a cruise ship or out in the desert. Maybe it was holding your baby for the first time. Perhaps it was a sexual moment that remains the gold standard in your love life.

Really probe your memory. Come up with the ultimate in pleasant recall. Color in all the details. Think about every moment of the experience from the time it began to its completion. Surrender your consciousness completely to this recollection of pleasure. Work on painting a mind picture of the pleasure for yourself at least once every day, and repeat it as often during the day as possible. You might notice that the pleasure becomes more intense every time you think about it.

Now, every time you conjure up that pleasant thought, give your right earlobe a gentle tug. You will begin to associate the tug with the pleasurable feeling. Soon the tug at the earlobe will be enough to remind you of the pleasant memory. The tug will make it easier to flood your thoughts with wonderful sensations. Finally the tug will be all it takes to make you feel great.

You can use this newly acquired, satisfying response to help with your weight loss efforts. Every time you start to think about forbidden foods, give a tug. When you're at a party with tables laden with treats, give a tug. Any time you're tempted to eat foods not permitted on the program, give a tug and start those pleasant associations flowing.

The time will surely come, and sooner than you might imagine possible, that you'll replace thoughts of food with thoughts of a completely different nature. As others indulge in their cakes and candies, you'll plunge into your pleasurable mental fantasy. No one need know what is going on in your mind. And all the while, you'll be farther along the road to permanent weight control.

Support Strategy 6: Realize You're in Good Company

It's part of human nature, when we are faced with a regrettable event, to ask, "Why me?" Being on a diet evokes that kind of thought from time to time, and it can involve feelings that range from mild perplexity to bitterness and resentment. "Why can't I eat those candies like my friends do?" "Why must I forego baked goods?" "Why can't I eat whatever I like without worrying about weight?" "Why me?"

Well, it's time to put things into their proper perspective. Just about everyone has to control some aspect of diet. Take a look around you and you'll see that it's not only you who has to be careful. For openers, estimates state that up to one in nine Americans is an alcoholic. Alcoholics' very lives are threatened by their inability to consume alcoholic beverages safely. The only way to control the condition is to abstain completely from alcohol for life.

Then there are the many sufferers of food allergies and sensitivities. Some people cannot tolerate the lactose in milk. Drinking even a glass of it can lead to severe gastric symptoms. Others develop skin rashes from eating foods such as strawberries or tomatoes. The list of food sensitivities and their medical consequences have filled volumes.

But, you might interrupt, what about my friend who eats like a horse and never gains a pound? She eats anything and everything. While it's true that there are exceptions to every rule, closer examination usually reveals that the rule still applies. If a person consumes more calories than can be burned, weight will eventually and inevitably be gained. That friend may be doing extensive exercise you're not aware of or dieting except when with friends or limiting herself in ways you're not seeing. Perhaps she *is* blessed with a strong metabolism. For whatever reason, you are not!

You have plenty of company in terms of limiting the food in your diet. You are *not* the lone victim you sometimes feel yourself to be.

Support Strategy 7: Celebrate Special Occasions Your Way

Is there a special celebration coming up? Birthdays, anniversaries, graduations, religious holidays, Halloween, and the holiday season from Thanksgiving to New Year's Eve are notorious food extravaganzas. The temptation is to say, "Oh well, it's just this once. One meal won't hurt."

On the face of it, that kind of thinking does seem reasonable. The problem is that "just this once" tends to apply to so many food-related situations during the year. Take another look at the list above. You can probably add a few more special occasions that apply to your own life. If you treat them all as "just this once," before you know it you'll be lapsing from your diet on a regular basis.

Many people refuse to begin a diet between Thanksgiving and New Year's Day. Then they make a resolution to lose all the weight gained during that long period of eating huge quantities of highly caloric foods. Other people say they can't start dieting until after their birthdays or after their vacations or until after other special occasions they've marked on the calendar. Pretty soon they've eliminated the entire year! For some people, there's *no* good time to begin to change the eating patterns that lead to and maintain overweight.

Any time is a good time to start dieting, especially on this program, because any time worth celebrating is worth highlighting with a commitment to future health and happiness. The forgone foods are a small sacrifice to make to achieve permanent weight loss.

Get out your calendar right now and mark all those times in the coming months and throughout the year when food temptations will be the strongest. The saying "Forewarned is forearmed" applies here. Start planning your strategies now so you won't be caught off guard when those special occasions come up.

What can you do to celebrate that has nothing to do with food? If you traditionally bake platters of cookies or gift boxes of fruitcake for Christmas presents, plan to make other kinds of gifts. How about homemade Christmas tree ornaments or floral arrangements? Scan through some magazines for specific suggestions and instructions.

Rather than going to a fancy restaurant to mark a birthday or an anniversary, why not get reservations for the theater or for a concert? Such outings would be far more special and out of the ordinary than another meal, no matter how expensive.

If you are invited to a party at a friend's home, be sure the friend knows that you won't be eating the foods offered. Be assertive about this. And then to weaken the temptations, have your meal before you go to the party.

On Halloween this year, eliminate the temptation to sample goodies bought for trick-or-treaters by giving out nonfood items. Replace candies with coins, gift certificates, or trinkets. You'll also be doing a favor for the parents of the children, who would probably prefer such treats to tooth-decaying sweets.

Thanksgiving is a time of gorging. The U.S. Department of Agriculture once calculated that, given the standard fare of turkey and all the trimmings, the average American male will consume up to 7,500 calories at one seating. But even a lapse far less dramatic than that can knock you out of ketosis and off your weight loss program. Yet that same Thanksgiving dinner can provide the very foods you want while following this program. Select your 4 ounces of turkey breast, a lettuce salad, and some spinach or another permitted vegetable. Declare yourself thankful that, in the face of abundance, you've decided to love yourself enough to pass it by. You might even enjoy feeling just a little smug about your demonstration of self-control. You are in control, and the rewards are so worth it!

Support Strategy 8: Keep Busy

If you've ever wanted to get involved with a hobby, this is the time to start. For those intent on changing their dietary habits, the old Puritan saying, "The devil finds work for idle hands," holds true. If your mind and hands aren't otherwise occupied, they can too easily be persuaded to fill the void with food.

It's pretty difficult to eat a pint of ice cream while doing needlepoint. (And needlework is not only for women. Professional football player Rosey Grier made his love of needlepoint well known.) You might renew some pleasant childhood memories. When was the last time you built a model airplane or painted a picture? What was your special enjoyment?

Take a trip to the local toy or hobby store and see if any of the items there appeal to you. Don't hesitate to select something that appears to be a child's toy: a wood-burning set or watercolors or modeling clay. Not only will these help you keep your mind and hands off food, but they might also prove to be wonderful ways to help you relax from the tensions of the day.

Consider also how you might be able to spend some of your spare time with others who need and would greatly appreciate your help. Think about doing some volunteer work at a children's hospital or a home for the elderly. Talk with your religious advisor or local volunteer centers about how you can help in the community. You'll feel good about your contribution, you'll eliminate many moments of temptation, and, if you have a tendency to do so, you'll stop feeling sorry for yourself.

Support Strategy 9: Be Prepared for When You Reach a Plateau

There comes a time in the life of all dieters, even those following this medically and scientifically superior approach, when they reach that puzzling dreaded stage known as a plateau, when even though they've done and are doing everything they're supposed to do, their weights stay the same. If it hasn't happened to you yet, it will. So it's best to be prepared to cope with this phenomenon.

The first thing to understand is that weight does not come off in a linear manner, with exactly the same number of pounds lost each day and each week. The first few days of any weight loss program will provide the greatest loss in pounds, largely because retained water weight is the first to go. From that point until goal weight is achieved, there will be peaks and valleys of loss.

Over the course of a week women typically lose 2 or 3 pounds and men 4 pounds, depending on the degree of overweight and physical activity. A given week might pass, however, when no weight loss occurs. That's why we suggest weighing yourself only weekly during weight loss. Weighing on a daily basis can be frustrating because of those peaks and valleys.

The most common cause of a plateau in weight loss is fluid retention, which women are more prone to than men. If the urine tests for ketones remain positive, then the failure to lose weight can be attributed to fluid retention and not to increased carbohydrate calories. Because you are still burning fat during a plateau and replacing it with an equivalent in water weight in nonfat areas, your clothes will feel looser. This is good reason to continue your body measurements through the period of weight loss. If the plateau is the result of not sticking with the program, which will take you out of ketosis, review your daily food intake in your diet diary. Perhaps a few more carbohydrates have slipped into your diet. If so, make the necessary corrections. This is why maintaining a food diary is so important.

During a plateau you can eliminate another pound or two by practicing the technique of diuresis of recumbency, described in Chapter 5.

The plateau is a time to renew your commitment and resolve to make permanent weight loss a reality. It's *not* the time to give up. The plateau is a normal, natural part of weight loss, and it will pass. How fast it will pass depends largely on your attitude and approach.

Support Strategy 10: Cope with Stress

Stress is an inherent part of dieting. The better you are at defusing that stress, the more successful you will be in your weight loss efforts. If you feel somewhat irritable because you miss some of your old favorite foods, even though you're not hungry, you're no different from anyone else who has gone on the program before you. It's a natural reaction to miss the foods you love to eat. Those foods have been an integral part of your life, but remember that now you're trying to change your lifestyle for the better.

Think of people you've known who have quit smoking cigarettes. With dieting and quitting smoking, one feels as if one is giving up a "best friend." Certain foods or cigarettes were always there to help you celebrate when things were good or console you when things were bad. It's tough to say good-bye to these friends, even though we know they're not good for us.

Just as one can predict that the person who quits smoking will get through the state of withdrawal, we know that the dieter will learn to cope with the loss of certain foods. However, in the meantime, you're still feeling stress, and knowing why or that it will eventually go away may not make you feel any better right now. There are two things you can do to lessen stressful moments.

Exercise has proved time and again to be effective in reducing diet-related stress. Not only is physical activity a substitute for eating, but it also has a relaxing, tranquilizing effect. Review the amount of activity you're getting each day, and see if you couldn't step up that level.

Sleep is always important for good physical and mental health, but it's even more important when you're under any kind of stress. A restful night's sleep from the special sedative trazodone can give you the energy and vitality to face the next day with renewed commitment to the weight loss program.

Relaxation techniques are essential components of a successful weight loss program. Are you taking the time each day to pursue a relaxed state? Remember, relaxing isn't a matter of collapsing in front of the television set at night. Whether it's yoga, meditation, hobbies, or other relaxing activities, relaxation techniques can greatly enhance the quality of your life. You owe yourself the twenty minutes or so a day that it takes to achieve a relaxed, stress-free state.

Support Strategy 11: Don't Be Afraid to Be Thin

Some people can become their own enemies, especially in the late stages of weight loss. After being insulated and protected by layers of fat for many years, they begin to have doubts about really wanting to shed that system of defense and give up their old familiar selves.

One patient had been severely overweight for all her teenage years and into early adulthood. She had never learned to deal with the attentions of men, since they seldom approached her. Suddenly, now that she was losing weight, all that was changing, and she was afraid. Her immediate response was to gain the weight back. But with the help of her brother, who accompanied her to dances and parties until she was able to cope on her own, she overcame her fear.

Others fear obesity is an excuse for not getting ahead in their careers. What if the weight is lost and the promotion still doesn't come along? Such fears may well undermine the weight loss effort.

Trying to hide under protective layers of fat is like covering your eyes so as not to see the negative aspects of life and missing the positive aspects as well. Life is too rich to hide from it. Any time you begin to doubt yourself or your ability to live happily as a slender person, think again about all the reasons why you're a lovable person. It's not that you'll be more lovable when you lose the weight; you'll still be the same old you underneath, but with more confidence and self-esteem. And remember, you *weren't* happy being overweight.

You'll have to cope with receiving compliments. You'll have to deal with being treated equally with others, not adversely or patronizingly because of your overweight. You may have to learn a few new skills along the way. But it's a great new life waiting for you to enjoy. Love yourself enough to grab every moment of happiness.

Support Strategy 12: Recognize the Traits That Predict Success

"Quitting cigarettes is easy—I've done it dozens of times." That old joke can be told about weight loss, too. The trick is not just losing weight, but keeping that weight off permanently.

There are certain personality traits that can predict failure in maintaining weight loss. Those most likely to regain lost weight, research has shown us, are men and women who demonstrate anxiety, avoidance of monotony, and a low degree of socialization. But those traits can be reversed, and, in doing so, you can greatly improve your chances for success.

To lessen anxiety, one must concentrate on those things that can promote relaxation, such as sufficient exercise, a good night's sleep, and specific relaxation activities.

Few people enjoy monotonous routines, but one can compensate for monotony in some things by substituting other activities at other times. For example, one might say that it's monotonous to be unable to break the meal plan routine by deciding at the moment to have ice cream or cheesecake for dessert. But if sufficient motivation and alternative activities are present, such feelings can be overcome. Your walks and new hobby can introduce much variety and spontaneity into your life.

Overweight men and women frequently have not learned social skills. It's difficult to say whether weight was the cause or the effect, the chicken or the egg. But one can make active efforts to become more social. For best results, such efforts should be gradual.

The best way to meet others with interests in common is to get involved in activities related to your own interests. Do you enjoy theater? Join a local drama group. Do you like modern art? Do some volunteer work at a museum. There are many people out there in the world who would enjoy your company. Volunteer work can help you feel involved and gradually more confident.

If none of these traits applies to you, we're certain that you'll lose weight and maintain that loss successfully for years and years to come. But if any trait is part of your personality, you can make some changes now. It will help in your efforts at weight loss, and it will enrich your entire life.

Support Strategy 13: Handle Your Anger

If you are the person primarily responsible for preparing food in your home, you might begin to feel some anger and resentment toward those who eat the foods you prepare when you personally can't. These feelings can result in tense family relations and possibly abandoning the diet. Both consequences are undesirable, so steps have to be taken to offset hostile emotions.

After the Christmas/Hanukkah holidays, one patient was fit to be tied. She was angry at "having" to cook all the foods she could not eat. "Next year I'm going to Las Vegas," she said. It's not always possible to "run away from home," but it may be possible to abdicate at least some responsibility in the kitchen. If your family is willing to do so, why not encourage them to eat some meals out in restaurants? Or perhaps they could, at least while you're in the weight loss phase, order some of their meals from take-out establishments. This might also be a good opportunity to teach others in the family a bit of responsibility for themselves. Even the youngest child can take a role in food preparation, serving, and cleanup.

In any case, the first thing to do when feeling anger or resentment about having to prepare foods for your family members is to have a frank discussion with them. Tell them that you understand the changes may be difficult for them, but also explain the importance of this diet to you. Success can mean enhanced health and happiness for the rest of your life. It may involve some changes in their routines and expectations, but aren't you worth such a small sacrifice?

Support Strategy 14: Don't Let Loved Ones Sabotage You

There are people out there ready and willing to sabotage your efforts at weight loss. The closer you get to your goal weight, the more temptations they seem to come up with, along with what they believe to be good reasons for you to eat the foods you've been trying to avoid.

The best possible defense against these well-meaning individuals is to know their lines of persuasion in advance. Then you won't be surprised when you hear them, and you'll be able to come up with counterarguments.

Get ready to hear . . .

"But just this one little piece of cake won't hurt."
"But I don't think you're heavy. *You* don't have to lose weight.
    You're perfect the way you are. Eat!"
"Try this chocolate mousse. I made it with you in mind."
"What's wrong? Don't you like the food?"

"I read that this brand is OK for dieters."

"Maybe you should quit that diet. You're getting too thin. Do you want to be skinny?"

"Haven't you been on that diet long enough?"

"Some people are *born* to be skinny, some heavy. You can't change your genes. Don't bother trying."

"Lots of heavy people live to be a hundred."

"It's your birthday. Why not splurge a little?"

"Go ahead and have some. You can always go back to the diet tomorrow."

"I don't think you should give up *all* your favorites."

"When you really miss foods, you should have just a taste to get you through."

"You're not feeling well, and they say, 'Feed a cold.' So enjoy this chicken soup I made just for you."

"Have some cake. It'll calm your nerves."

"It's not *natural* to eat so little."

"This candy is good for diabetics."

"We love you, Mom. We don't care if you're heavy. You won't be the same if you lose weight."

"I love you, dear. That's why I married you even though you were heavy. I just adore cuddling you. Won't you stop this dieting?"

These are the kinds of comments you can expect to hear from friends, relatives, and loved ones. Only *you* know how much you want to lose that weight. Don't let *anyone* stand in the way of your future health and happiness. Even if some people seem disappointed when you don't join them in eating certain foods, they will respect you for it.

Support Strategy 15: Know What to Do When You Fail

We'd like to think that everyone who begins this program will continue straight along until reaching goal weight and then maintain that loss for the rest of their lives, never once falling off the wagon. But we know that's just not to be. There's a good chance that you will slip. There's nothing wrong with falling down. But there's no reason in the world not to get right back up again.

Lest you think you're different from everyone else in the world, let us reassure you that many others have slipped and fallen before you. Those who respond by abandoning the program altogether tend to have in common a general lack of self-confidence and self-respect. Some, after giving in to temptation and gaining weight, look at themselves in the mirror with disgust. "I knew I couldn't do it," they say. "I don't deserve any better in life. There's no point in going on with this. I'm just a fat slob and no one cares about me anyway. Why should I care? I might as well eat."

That scenario has been played and replayed again and again. You very well may have some of the same feelings if you splurge and gain back some of the weight you lost. But you have to fight those feelings.

Everyone has little failures. No one is perfect. We do ourselves more damage by punishing ourselves for failing than by the failures themselves. So forgive yourself. Do so because you love yourself enough to get up and start again.

If you've brought some carbohydrates into the house, throw them out or give them away. Get right back on the program and into ketosis. Be forewarned, however, that it may be more difficult to reenter the state of ketosis than it was to get into it initially. It might take a day or two more. But you can and will get back into ketosis.

There's a saying that every millionaire went broke once or twice before making his or her ultimate fortune. The same applies to those trying to lose weight. Failing once or twice may just be paving the way for success. Have faith in yourself. Love yourself. You can do it, and you will.

Support Strategy 16: Prepare for Parties

We all enjoy going to parties and get-togethers, but the temptations of the buffet table can spoil the fun. Before going to such events, make sure to eat some substantial low carbohydrate foods to deliberately spoil your appetite. By the time you arrive at the party, you won't be hungry and you'll easily pass on those treats that could otherwise undermine your diet.

Strategy 17: Make Plans for Holidays

It's true that most of the holiday seasons seem to be celebrated with sugary foods. Instead of giving in to those high carbohydrate diet destroyers, thinks of some alternatives. On Easter, make plenty of brightly colored hard-boiled eggs to replace the chocolate ones. Around Halloween, keep bowls of little trinkets and toys around for the trick-or-treaters. On Valentine's Day, stick with flowers and forget the candies, and be sure to tell your loved ones your preference for gifts. Passover is the celebration when the children of Israel were finally released by Pharaoh. The song "Let My People Go" told this story. For Passover, remember that by reducing your insulin you can liberate your fat from bondage. (Let My Stored Fat Go!) Celebrate Thanksgiving by being grateful for the weight loss you've been enjoying, and sticking with the turkey and salad and other low carbohydrate foods.

Chapter 11

INSULIN CONTROL FOODS AND RECIPES

One of the great advantages of the dietary aspects of this program is the wide variety of foods it allows you every day. In Chapter 6 we outlined a full two weeks of meal plans. You'll notice that you won't repeat any of the entrees, except for the occasional use of leftovers for lunchtime convenience. Using the recipes in this chapter, you'll be able to create week after week of delicious menu plans. Seek the widest variety of foods possible, and don't let yourself slip into a rut of preparing foods the same way over and over. Give all the recipes a try. By the time you determine which are your favorites, you'll be well on your way to a slender new self.

Note: We have deliberately not included a breakdown of calories, fat, protein, and carbohydrates in the recipes for this program. The reason is simple: We want you to be able to follow the program without worrying about calories and to learn to determine your own nutritional needs.

Spend some time with the lists of foods provided to acquaint yourself with their nutrition analyses. Then you'll know at a glance if foods in question will be appropriate for you, whether you're in the weight loss, stabilization, or maintenance phase of the program.

Bon appétit!

BREAKFAST DISHES

There's no more traditional breakfast food than the egg, which starts the day for people in countries all over the world. Because eggs contain a wealth of nutrients, are a marvelous source of protein, are low in fat and calories, and contain no carbohydrates, they are an excellent choice as a part of your weight loss program.

Of course, eggs do have a high cholesterol content, with more than 200 milligrams in one large egg. But many individuals can eat an egg a day without any elevation in cholesterol levels. If you don't know your cholesterol level, it's a good idea to have it checked; your physician can tell you how. If your cholesterol level is normal, you can continue to enjoy your daily egg. If it's slightly elevated, your physician may advise you to eat only two or three weekly. If your cholesterol level is quite elevated, you should eliminate whole eggs from your diet.

All the egg's cholesterol is found in the yolk; there is none in the white. If you are advised to eliminate whole eggs, you can use two whites instead of one egg. There are also a number of egg substitutes, which are made from egg whites and contain no cholesterol. These can be used to make scrambled eggs that can scarcely be distinguished from fresh eggs.

If you aren't already familiar with the many ways eggs can be prepared, here are a few of them.

Poached

In a small saucepan bring water to a gentle boil. Crack an egg into a small dish. Swirl the water in the pan into a little whirlpool and gently slide the egg into the center of the whirlpool. Cook for 2 to 3 minutes. Remove with a slotted spoon.

Makes 1 serving

Soft Cooked

Place an egg in a small saucepan of cold water, enough to completely cover the egg, and bring to a boil. Boil gently for 3½ minutes for the classic soft-cooked egg, a bit less for a runnier egg, and a bit more for a firmer one.

Makes 1 serving

Hard Cooked

Place an egg in a small saucepan of cold water, enough to completely cover the egg, and bring to a boil. Cover the pan and turn off the heat. Let stand for 20 minutes. Remove the egg and hold it under cold running water for about 30 seconds. You might want to make several hard-cooked eggs at once, so you will have some to peel as needed.

Makes 1 serving

Sunnyside Up

This classic egg dish is usually made with butter or oil, but this version eliminates most of those fat grams and calories. Spray some butter-flavored vegetable spray on a nonstick pan. Crack an egg into the pan over medium heat and fry until the white is no longer translucent and the yolk is done to your taste.

Makes 1 serving

Scrambled

The trick to making perfect scrambled eggs is to beat them lightly in a bowl prior to cooking. Spray a nonstick pan with vegetable spray and start to heat. Pour the beaten egg into the pan. Cook over low heat, scrambling, until set. You may substitute one of the brands of cholesterol-free egg substitutes. For flavor variety, add a few drops of vanilla, almond, or orange extract while scrambling.

Makes 1 serving

Basted

This delicious variation on the sunnyside-up egg is a cross between a fried and a poached egg. Proceed as for a sunnyside-up egg, but after putting the egg in the pan, pour 1 tablespoon of water over the egg and cover the pan. For those watching cholesterol, try using only the whites of two eggs instead of a whole egg.

Makes 1 serving

Deviled

Slice hard-cooked eggs in half lengthwise, and place the yolks in a bowl. For each yolk add 1 teaspoon of nonfat milk and a dash each of paprika, onion powder, dry mustard, minced chives, and salt.

Mash the yolks. Fill the egg whites with the yolk mixture, and sprinkle with paprika and chives.

1 egg per serving

Elliott's "Made in Spain" Omelet

2 tablespoons olive oil
2–3-inch segment of Soyrizo sausage, removed from casing and made into patties
2 large eggs (or equivalent egg substitute), beaten
6 sugar-cube-size chunks of Spanish Iberico cheese

Heat the olive oil in a medium frying pan until hot. Add sausage patties. When the patties are brown on one side, flip them and add the beaten eggs and cheese around the patties. Lower the heat and cover. When the eggs begin to set and the cheese begins to melt, fold the mixture in half, cover, and cook until done.

Makes 1 serving

Elliott's Low Carb Pancakes

1 cup almond flour
2 eggs
¼ cup water (for puffier pancakes, use sparkling water)
2 tablespoons oil
¼ teaspoon salt
1 tablespoon sweetener
Dash baking powder
Dash cinnamon
Few drops of vanilla extract
Canola oil *or* cooking spray
Sugar free Maple syrup

Combine all ingredients. Drop by the ladleful onto a medium-hot pan coated with canola oil or cooking spray. Top with maple syrup.

Makes four large or eight small pancakes

PHYTOSTEROLS: A NEW WAY OF FIGHTING CHOLESTEROL

Thanks to a massive public education program sponsored by the National Institutes of Health in cooperation with the leading medical organizations, practically everyone realizes that elevated cholesterol levels in the blood present a major risk factor for heart disease. Both saturated fat and dietary cholesterol in foods tend to raise levels of cholesterol in the blood. Not surprisingly, then, sales of eggs, liver, and other cholesterol-rich foods have dropped precipitously. Compared to those of twenty years ago, consumption rates of eggs have plummeted by more than 50 percent. Happily, there is now a way to enjoy all those foods once again—by blocking the absorption of cholesterol with a plant substance known as *phytosterol.*

Cholesterol is a member of the chemical family called sterols, which are present in every animal tissue. Cholesterol is an animal sterol. Plants also contain sterols, which are termed *phytosterols*—the yin and yang of nature.

You may remember that many years ago dietitians condemned shellfish for having very high levels of cholesterol. Those early measurements were totally inaccurate because they were counting not only cholesterol but also the phytosterols from the plants those animals ate. Shellfish are the vegetarians of the sea. In truth, shellfish have the lowest cholesterol content of any animal food, a third of that found in chicken breast, for example. That makes all shellfish—scallops, clams, oysters, crab, lobster, shrimp—perfect for those following our weight loss program. All shellfish are virtually devoid of fat and very low in calories. But those early measurement devices could not tell the difference between cholesterol and phytosterol.

Well, neither can your body! Cholesterol is absorbed in the first one-third of your intestine by cell receptors that pass it along into the bloodstream. Those receptor sites can't discern between cholesterol and phytosterols, and they'll fill up on whichever happens to be available. The phytosterols, however, are not absorbed into the bloodstream. They simply block the receptor sites for a period of time. The wonderful part of this fluke of physiology is that if those cellular docking sites are filled with phytosterols, there's no room for absorption of cholesterol, which simply passes along the intestine and is ultimately excreted.

Phytosterols are found in all plants, from fruits to vegetables to oils. Because they are soluble in fat, as cholesterol is, the principal concentration of plant sterols is in vegetable oils of all kinds. However, plant sterols cause these oils to be cloudy, and food manufacturers remove them to provide the clear product that consumers prefer. Thus, there is no readily available source of concentrated phytosterols in our diet.

Interestingly, the Japanese make oil from rice bran, which they remove to produce the white rice that they prefer. But, they leave the clouding phytosterols in rice oil, which may be one reason the Japanese have a low rate of heart disease.

The term *phytosterols* is generic and includes all plant sterols. The principal phytosterols in nature are beta-sitosterol, stigmasterol, and campesterol. Sitosterol is the most potent phytosterol for blocking the absorption of cholesterol. That discovery was first made in the late 1940s.

Research with phytosterols continued through the 1970s and into the 1980s. Probably the most definitive study came from the laboratories of Fred Mattson and Scott Grundy at the University of California at San Diego. They fed hospitalized patients scrambled eggs and sitosterol and found that the phytosterol blocked the absorption of cholesterol, resulting in reduced cholesterol levels in the blood.

Often researchers used phytosterols as a general cholesterol-lowering agent rather than to specifically block the absorption of dietary cholesterol in a particular meal. This meant that at one meal there would be more phytosterol than needed, when not much cholesterol was present in the foods; while at other times there would not be enough to block the absorption of all the cholesterol available. Even so, studies showed total cholesterol reductions of 12 percent on average.

Why aren't phytosterols more popular? One reason is lack of publicity. No major company produces phytosterols. As a plant substance, no one can hold an exclusive patent, and the money is in patented products. So, while they are available, companies can't afford to advertise. Interestingly, research in Finland published in the *New England Journal of Medicine* in 1995 showed a 10 percent cholesterol reduction from phytosterols blended into margarine. Today that margarine is a big seller in Finland, even though the price is ten times that of regular spreads.

To be effective, one has to counteract cholesterol with phytosterols on at least a one-to-one basis, assuming a high-quality phytosterol preparation. Since one egg contains about 220 milligrams of cholesterol, it takes at least that much phytosterol to block its absorption.

There's no question about the efficacy of phytosterols in blocking cholesterol from foods eaten and in lowering the cholesterol level in the blood. Research by some of the world's most prestigious universities has been published in major medical journals. Most recently, a review article showing the benefits of phytosterols was published as a scientific advisory to physicians in *Circulation*, the official publication of the American Heart Association.

But are they safe? Phytosterols are one of the safest substances you could possibly ingest. To quote Scott Grundy at the University of Texas Southwestern Medical Center, "Phytosterols have the added advantage of causing little or no side effects."

Today there is no reason why even the most heart-healthy person, even if he or she has a tendency toward elevated cholesterol levels, should avoid eggs and other cholesterol-rich foods such as liver. The phytosterols can completely block cholesterol while allowing us to enjoy those foods and benefit from all their nutrients.

You can find phytosterols in many health food stores and pharmacies. Examples of supplements that contain phytosterols are Nature Made CholestOff, Twinlab Cholesterol Success, and Futurebiotics Cholesterol Balance.

Take one 400-milligram tablet with each meal containing any amount of cholesterol to achieve a cholesterol-lowering effect. To block cholesterol in foods particularly rich with it, take two tablets thirty minutes prior to the meal, along with a big glass of water.

While egg substitutes can make an adequate omelet, nothing can take the place of real eggs. With all the potential preparation methods, you just never get tired of them. Similarly, liver is a wonderful food, containing very little fat yet providing high-quality protein and an array of nutrients, especially iron and vitamin B_{12}. Enjoy both eggs and liver as part of this program.

BOUILLON

You'll come to rely on bouillon as you follow this weight control program. It's low in fat, carbohydrate, and calories, yet flavorful and satisfying. When you'd like a pick-me-up in the middle of the afternoon, reach for a steaming cup of chicken, beef, or vegetable bouillon. When sautéing or stir-frying various foods, use a tablespoon of bouillon instead of oil. You will also use bouillon in a number of recipes.

Several canned and instant bouillons (powders and cubes) are available. Choose the best ones by reading their nutrient labels. Most canned beef bouillons (or broths, the terms are interchangeable) contain just 1 gram of carbohydrate and only 16 calories per 8-ounce serving prepared according to label directions. There is more variation among the instant bouillon mixes. Weight Watchers packets, when mixed with water to make 6 ounces of bouillon, contain 1 gram of carbohydrate and 8 calories. Romanoff MBT brand supplies 12 calories and 2 grams of carbohydrate. It is a slight difference, but it can add up.

VEGETABLE DISHES

We encourage you to have vegetables every day on this program. Vegetables are a low fat, low calorie, nutrient-packed component of a balanced diet for everyone. Start now to get into the good habit of selecting a variety of vegetables to enjoy regularly. Remember that a serving size of vegetables is ½ cup cooked or 1 cup raw.

While you can simply open a can of green beans or defrost some frozen broccoli, you'll find the program much more enjoyable and healthful if you use fresh vegetables. Try some you haven't had in a while or have never tried.

Although some nutrients are lost in canned vegetables, they can come in handy when you're in a hurry. Frozen vegetables contain more nutrients than canned, and you can measure out a serving for yourself and return the rest to the freezer. Try perking up the flavor of frozen and canned vegetables by adding snippets of fresh herbs such as basil and dill.

Properly prepared steamed or boiled vegetables are delicious, but even the most health-conscious dieter can get tired of them in their

plain states day after day. However, the alternative is not to add butter or cream or other highly caloric sauces. Rather, explore the possibilities of using fresh and dried herbs and spices. More than ever
before, fresh herbs can be found in most supermarkets. Simply adding a fresh herb to a fresh vegetable can transform a simple dish into
a taste experience. Whether using fresh or dried herbs, start with
small amounts and increase until you reach your own taste preference. Don't overdo it. You can use only one flavoring or mix them,
according to your taste. Garlic and ginger, for example, go particularly well together, providing an oriental flavor when used with a
dash of soy sauce. Here is a list of vegetables and some herbs and
spices that go particularly well with them.

Asparagus: basil, garlic, sesame seed
Beans: savory, basil, chili powder, nutmeg, sage, dill
Broccoli: mace, oregano
Cabbage: dill, mace, oregano, caraway seeds
Cauliflower: chili powder, dill, nutmeg
Pea pods: marjoram, oregano, mint
Spinach: chervil, marjoram, nutmeg
Squash, winter: cloves, nutmeg
Turnips: dill, basil

Why limit yourself to the color and flavor of just one vegetable at
a time? Mix two or three vegetables to make terrific combinations.
Just make sure the total does not exceed the serving size of ½ cup
cooked or 1 cup raw. By keeping several kinds in the freezer, you
can mix to your heart's content. Here are a few combinations you
might like to try. Use your imagination to come up with some of
your own.

Brussels sprouts and carrot slices
Green cabbage and red cabbage
Onions, mushrooms, and broccoli
Pea pods, mushrooms, and water chestnuts
Cauliflower and broccoli florets

Following are some simple recipes and basic preparation methods
for a variety of vegetables.

Artichoke

Artichokes are a fun food. You'll enjoy picking the leaves off one at a time and scraping them between your teeth to get at the flesh. And when you've finished the succulent part of the leaves, you still have a couple of bites of the delicious artichoke bottom to savor. A serving of artichoke is half of one medium artichoke. Select artichokes that have tight rather than opened leaves.

To prepare, remove any discolored and small leaves at the base of the artichoke. Cut off the stem and the top of the globe. Snip off the tips of the leaves with scissors. Remove the small, pale inner leaves at the top of the globe. Scrape out all of the fuzzy choke below the inner leaves. Rinse and drop into a bowl of water with some lemon juice added until ready to cook. In a saucepan just large enough to hold the number of artichokes you are cooking, bring to a boil enough water to cover the artichokes. Add 1 teaspoon of lemon juice, 1 clove of garlic, and 1 teaspoon of salt. Add the artichokes and return to boil. Reduce heat and simmer uncovered for 30 to 40 minutes or until the leaves pull off easily. Drain and serve either hot or cold.

Asparagus Chinese Style

Asparagus is a treat just steamed or boiled, but for some variety try this dish with a Chinese flavor. Trim off the hard ends of the spears. Cut the asparagus on a diagonal into 1½-inch pieces to make ½ cup (3–4 stalks). Add ½ teaspoon of salt to 1 cup of water in a shallow pan. Bring water to a boil and add asparagus. Cook 5 to 7 minutes or until just tender to a fork. While the asparagus is cooking, make a sauce by combining 2 tablespoons chicken bouillon, 1 teaspoon soy sauce, a dash of ground ginger, and a dash of Chinese five-spice seasoning. Drain the asparagus, return it to the pan with the sauce, heat quickly, and serve.

Beans with Basil

Snap off the tips of fresh beans and slice into 1-inch pieces. Place in a small saucepan with 1 cup of cold, salted water for each 1 cup of raw beans. Bring to a boil. Add two or three basil leaves. Cook for 5 to 10 minutes. Drain and serve.

Bean Sprouts

Chinese cooking isn't the only place for bean sprouts. Try them with a number of dishes to add a distinctive crunch. In a medium-sized skillet, bring 2 tablespoons of chicken bouillon to a boil. Add 1 cup of bean sprouts per person. Cover and cook for just 2 minutes. Don't overcook.

Broccoli

The bright green color of properly prepared broccoli adds excitement to any plate of food. The trick is not to overcook it. Trim off leaves and cut off as much stalk as you wish. Cut into florets and place in a large skillet with a cover. Add 1 inch of cold salted water, bring to a boil, and cover. Cook approximately 3 minutes, until broccoli is fork tender and emerald green.

Brussels Sprouts

These little cabbages are a nice change of pace. Shop for the smallest ones you can find, with tight leaves. Trim off any excess stalk, and, if you have the patience, pierce the stalk end with the tip of a knife. Bring 1 inch of salted water to a boil in a shallow pan. Add the sprouts, bring to a boil, cover, and cook for about 10 minutes or until tender.

Cabbage

Prepare red cabbage, green cabbage, or some of both by shredding enough to fill 1 cup per person. In a pot large enough to accommodate the cabbage, bring ½ inch of salted water with 2 tablespoons of vinegar to a boil. Put in the cabbage, cover, and cook 8 to 10 minutes.

Cauliflower

One medium head of cauliflower comes out to about four servings. Remove the heavy stalk and leaves and cut into small florets. Bring 1 inch of salted water to a boil in a medium skillet. Place the cauliflower in the skillet, cover, and cook for about 20 minutes. Perk it up by serving with colorful strips of red pimento.

Chinese Pea Pods (Snow Peas)

These flat, bright green pods shouldn't wait for a Chinese meal. They make a wonderful accompaniment to any dinner. Snap off the ends and remove any strings. Bring 1 inch of salted water to a boil, add the pea pods, and cook for just 2 minutes so they're still crisp.

Spinach

Rinse a bunch of spinach thoroughly before you remove the binding ties. With a large knife cut the stems off at the base of the leaves. Fill the kitchen sink with water and swirl the spinach leaves around in it to remove any residual sand. Shake the spinach dry and place in a large pot with only the water clinging to its leaves. Use a stainless steel, enameled, or coated pot. Do not cook spinach in aluminum. Cover and cook over a medium-high heat for about 3 minutes.

Zucchini

This versatile vegetable can be eaten raw or cooked. Cut it raw into julienne strips or shred it to add to a salad. Slice it or cut it into chunks and boil for about 7 minutes in salted water. Cut a small zucchini in half lengthwise, place it 6 inches under the broiler, and broil 10 to 12 minutes or until fork tender.

Elliott's Faux Couscous with Onion and Mushrooms

1 whole cauliflower
½ medium onion, chopped
6–8 medium mushrooms, chopped

2 cloves garlic, minced
2 tablespoons olive oil
Salt to taste

Cut away as much of the cauliflower stalk as possible. Cut the cauliflower into small segments and pulse in food processor until the consistency is similar to couscous. Cook in a microwave-safe covered dish for 4 minutes. Sauté onion, mushrooms, and garlic in olive oil until onions are tender. Mix into the cauliflower. Salt to taste.

Makes 4 servings

Low Carb Lasagna

1 medium zucchini
Olive oil
2–3 cups pasta sauce (try to find low sugar sauce)
1 medium onion, chopped
3 cloves garlic, minced
1 cup mushrooms, sliced
2–3 turkey sausage links or patties
½ pound ground turkey
2 teaspoons Italian seasoning
Nonstick cooking spray
8 ounces ricotta cheese
2 cups grated mozzarella

Cut the zucchini into ¼-inch slices, drizzle with olive oil, and bake in a preheated 350°F oven until soft (about 10 minutes). Pour pasta sauce into a saucepan. Add onion, garlic, and mushrooms. Heat until warm. Heat a little olive oil in a skillet. Add turkey sausage and ground turkey. Brown. Stir in Italian seasoning. Drain any liquid from the pan and then add contents to the saucepan with the pasta sauce. Coat an 8-inch glass baking dish with nonstick spray. Cover the bottom of the dish with a layer of the pasta-sauce mixture. Top with ricotta, then mozzarella, and then zucchini. Repeat layers until the dish is full. Bake in a preheated 350°F oven for 20–30 minutes or until cheese melts and all of the layers are warm.

Makes 2 servings

Macaroni and Cheese

1 bag frozen cauliflower
Salt and pepper to taste
2 tablespoons cream cheese
1 small pat butter
Nonstick cooking spray
½ cup shredded cheese (Colby jack and cheddar)
½ cup shredded sharp cheddar

Boil the cauliflower until tender. Add salt and pepper to taste and stir in the cream cheese and butter. Pour into an 8-inch square baking dish coated with nonstick spray. Sprinkle with cheeses. Bake in a preheated 400°F oven for 20–30 minutes until cheese melts.

Makes 2 servings

FISH AND SHELLFISH

For the health- and weight-conscious eater, the ultimate entree is fish and shellfish. High in protein and low in fat, these foods are rapidly replacing beef and pork on the dinner table. If you haven't already jumped on the fish bandwagon, this is the perfect time to do so.

The freshness of fish and seafood is the all-important factor for taste. Fresh fish does not smell "fishy." The store itself should smell fresh and clean. Ask when the fish was received and what the freshest "catch of the day" is. On a whole fish, the eyes should be relatively clear and not sunken in. On fillets, be certain the skin hasn't begun to curl and that the flesh is moist. Ask the shopkeeper for advice on best quality, good buys, and cooking methods, and don't be afraid to try new varieties.

There's a simple rule when it comes to cooking fish. Regardless of the type or cut of fish, regardless of the method of cooking, cook for no more than ten minutes per 1-inch thickness of fish. Whether it's a whole fish or a fillet, measure the thickest part of the fish. *Most* fillets and steaks will be no more than 1 inch thick. This rule applies to broiling, grilling, and sautéing. When fish is combined with other ingredients and baked, it may take longer. Fish is considered done as soon as it has lost its translucent color. You do not want to overcook any type of fish or shellfish. In the past one was advised to cook until the flesh began to "flake," but most chefs today would consider this overdone. You want the fish to be moist and juicy.

You can enjoy a wide variety of fish prepared in many ways. To get you started, we've provided some favorite recipes. Fish may not be "brain food," but it certainly is a smart choice.

Baked Fish Fillet

4 ounces fish fillet (sea bass or snapper is excellent)
1 tablespoon chopped tomato
1 pinch each tarragon, dill weed, finely chopped chives

Rinse the fish well under cold running water; pat dry with paper towel. Place the fish in a glass or ceramic casserole dish and cover with chopped tomato and seasonings. Cover. Bake in a preheated 350°F oven for 15 minutes.

Makes 1 serving

Florentine Fish Fillet

4 ounces fish fillet
3 tablespoons chopped spinach
1 tablespoon chopped onion
1 pinch each thyme, salt, pepper

Rinse the fish well under cold running water; pat dry with paper towel. Place the fish in the middle of a 12-inch square of aluminum foil. Cover with the spinach, onion, and seasonings. Fold over the foil and seal tightly. Bake in a preheated 350°F oven for 10 to 12 minutes. Open immediately upon removal from oven to stop the cooking process.

Makes 1 serving

Chinese Fish Steak

Vegetable oil spray
½ teaspoon each finely chopped garlic and fresh ginger
1 teaspoon soy sauce
½ cup chicken bouillon
4 ounces fish steak (halibut, shark, tuna, swordfish)
3 tablespoons chopped mushrooms

In a small pan coated with vegetable oil spray, sauté garlic and ginger briefly. Do not let garlic brown. Add soy sauce and bouillon to pan, and heat to boiling. Transfer the bouillon mixture to a small casserole dish. Add the fish to the casserole and spread the mushrooms on top of it. Cover. Bake in a preheated 350°F oven for 15 to 20 minutes.

Makes 1 serving

Salmon in Court Bouillon

1 cup water
1 tablespoon lemon juice
2 bay leaves
6 peppercorns
1 garlic clove, quartered
3 slices onion
1 large sprig fresh dill
4 ounces salmon fillet or steak

Mix all the ingredients except the salmon in a casserole dish. Place the salmon in the mixture and arrange the sliced onion over it. Cover the dish with a sheet of waxed paper. Bake in a preheated 350°F oven for 20 minutes.

Makes 1 serving

Teriyaki Broiled Fish

1 tablespoon soy sauce
1 teaspoon lemon juice

1 garlic clove, finely minced
½ teaspoon finely minced fresh ginger
4 ounces fish fillet or steak (a firm-fleshed variety, such as
    salmon or shark)

Mix all the ingredients except the fish in a plastic food storage bag.
Place the fish in the bag and marinate for 30 minutes or longer. Place
the fish on a broiler tray or grill, and broil or grill for 10 minutes.

Makes 1 serving

New Orleans Creole Fillet

1 tablespoon each chopped tomato, onion, celery, green pepper
1 garlic clove, finely minced
1 tablespoon tomato juice
¼ teaspoon chili powder
4 ounces fish fillet (red snapper, grouper)

Mix all the ingredients except the fish in a casserole dish. Place the
fish in a dish and spoon the mixture over it. Cover. Bake in a preheated 350°F oven for 15 minutes.

Makes 1 serving

Indian Fish Curry

1 tablespoon each chopped onion, mushrooms, tomato
1 teaspoon lemon juice
1 teaspoon curry powder
4 ounces white fish fillet (cod, white fish, orange roughy)

Mix all the ingredients except the fish in a casserole dish. Place the
fish in the dish and spoon the mixture over it. Cover. Bake in a preheated 350°F oven for 15 minutes.

Makes 1 serving

Blackened Fish

2 tablespoons unprocessed bran
1 tablespoon Cajun Blackening Seasoning (see recipe on page
    199)
4 ounces fish fillet
2 tablespoons beaten egg *or* egg substitute
Vegetable oil spray

Mix the unprocessed bran with the Cajun Blackening Seasoning.
Dip the fish fillet first into the egg and then into the bran mixture to
coat it. Coat a pan with vegetable oil spray and heat on high heat.
Sauté the fillet for about 3 to 4 minutes on each side.

Makes 1 serving

Broiled Seafood Kebabs

2 tablespoons lemon juice
1 garlic clove, finely minced
½ teaspoon salt
¼ teaspoon pepper
4 ounces seafood (scallops, shrimp, fish chunks, or a mixture)
1 cup total raw vegetables (whole mushrooms, green pepper
    chunks, onions cut into quarters or eighths)

Mix lemon juice, garlic, salt, and pepper in a plastic food storage bag.
Add the seafood and vegetables, and marinate for 30 minutes or longer. Skewer seafood and vegetables alternately. Broil for 3 minutes
on one side. Turn and broil for another 2 minutes.

Note: This dish includes both the protein food and the vegetable for a
meal.

Makes 1 serving

This 'n' That Seafood Soup

This type of dish was the origin of bouillabaisse and cioppino. As
you purchase fish and shellfish and find an ounce of this and an
ounce of that left over, save these morsels in the freezer. Then when

you have enough for the recipe (or multiply it for the entire family), you'll have a treat!

½ cup water
1 teaspoon lemon juice
2 tablespoons chopped tomato
2 tablespoons chopped onion
1 pinch saffron
1 teaspoon salt
½ teaspoon pepper
4 ounces total seafood (shrimp, scallops, fish, crab, lobster)

Mix all the ingredients except the seafood in a pot and bring to a boil. Lower the heat, add the seafood, and cook 10 minutes at a slow simmer.

Makes 1 serving

Oriental Seafood Stir-Fry

3 tablespoons chicken bouillon
1 tablespoon oyster sauce
1 teaspoon soy sauce
1 garlic clove, finely minced
½ teaspoon finely minced fresh ginger
4 ounces seafood, cut into even-sized pieces (scallops, shrimp, crab, lobster, or a mixture)
1 cup total vegetables, cut into even-sized pieces (bean sprouts, water chestnuts, mushrooms, broccoli, Chinese cabbage)

Mix together 2 tablespoons of the chicken bouillon, oyster sauce, soy sauce, garlic, and ginger. Heat a large skillet or wok. Add the remaining tablespoon of chicken bouillon to the wok and quickly stir-cook the seafood and vegetables. Add the bouillon mixture and bring to a boil. Serve.

Note: This dish includes both the protein food and the vegetable for a meal.

Makes 1 serving

Broiled Shrimp and Scallops

1 tablespoon lemon juice
1 garlic clove, finely minced
1 tablespoon finely minced cilantro
2 ounces shrimp
2 ounces scallops

Mix lemon juice, garlic, and cilantro in a plastic food storage bag. Add the seafood and marinate for 30 minutes or longer. Grill or broil for 3 minutes on one side. Turn and broil for an additional 2 minutes.

Makes 1 serving

Salmon or Tuna Salad Sandwich

4 ounces canned salmon or tuna, packed in water
1 tablespoon each finely chopped onion, celery, green pepper
½ teaspoon dill weed
1 teaspoon lemon juice
½ teaspoon salt
1 teaspoon reduced-calorie mayonnaise
2 large lettuce leaves or 1 piece of low carb bread

Drain the tuna or salmon. Remove any skin and bones from the salmon. Mix all the ingredients except the lettuce leaves or bread. If using lettuce leaves spread the mixture on one; cover with the second leaf to form a sandwich. Or use low carb bread to make an open-face sandwich.

Makes 1 serving

Salmon Patties

4 ounces canned salmon, packed in water
1 egg white
2 tablespoons unprocessed bran
1 tablespoon finely chopped onion
1 teaspoon minced parsley

1 teaspoon lemon juice
¼ teaspoon salt
¼ teaspoon pepper
Vegetable oil spray

Drain the salmon and remove any skin and bones. Mix all the ingredients together (except cooking spray) and form two patties. Coat a pan with vegetable oil spray and heat on moderate heat. Sauté the patties until crispy on the outside.

Makes 1 serving

Salmon Chowder

Here's a recipe to use all those scraps of salmon you have left over from other recipes. Freeze them until you have enough to make this delicious meal in a bowl.

1 cup total vegetables, diced (carrots, parsnips, turnips)
1 cup chicken bouillon
1 tablespoon chopped onion
¼ teaspoon salt
¼ teaspoon pepper
1 dash hot pepper sauce
4 ounces salmon chunks (skin removed)

Cook the vegetables in seasoned bouillon for 10 minutes. Add the salmon. Cook 10 additional minutes.

Note: This dish includes both the protein food and the vegetable for a meal.

Makes 1 serving

Oven "Fried" Scallops

The main reason most of us like deep-fried foods is that wonderful crunch when we take a bite. This recipe duplicates the crunch and flavor without the fat and calories. You can do this same recipe with shrimp or fish fillets. For variety, change the seasonings in the bran mixture. You might try some of the commercial seasoning mixtures, such as lemon-herb.

2 tablespoons unprocessed bran
¼ teaspoon each salt, paprika, ground pepper, garlic powder
3 ounces bay or sea scallops
1 beaten egg or egg substitute
Vegetable oil spray
Lemon wedges

Mix the bran with the seasonings in a plastic food storage bag. Dip the scallops into the beaten egg in a bowl. Drop a few scallops at a time into the bag and shake until coated. Place on a cookie sheet and spray with the vegetable oil spray. Bake in a preheated 400°F oven for 10 minutes. Serve with a squeeze of lemon.

Makes 1 serving

Crispy Breaded Fish Fillets

2 tablespoons unprocessed bran
¼ teaspoon each paprika, salt, pepper, onion powder
4 ounces fish fillet without skin
2 tablespoons beaten egg *or* egg substitute
Vegetable oil spray

Mix the seasonings with the bran. Dip the fish first into the egg and then into the seasoned bran to coat it. Sauté 8 to 10 minutes in a pan coated with vegetable oil spray.

Makes 1 serving

Steaming Seafood

Have you ever wondered why fish tastes so fresh and moist when served in Chinese or Japanese restaurants? It's because they steam their seafood. This technique is remarkably simple, yet most people don't attempt it in their own kitchens. And, if you're in a hurry, there's no faster way to prepare food. Just toss a 4-ounce serving into the steamer and set the timer; in minutes it's ready to eat. All you need are a large pot or frying pan with a cover and a steaming rack. You can pick up a rack in any housewares department. Buy a large enough rack to fit into a large pot or pan.

Put 1 inch of water into the bottom of the pot. Place the rack in the pot; the water should not reach the surface of the rack on which the food will rest. Bring the water to a boil to produce steam in the pot. Place the food directly on the rack or put it in a plate on the rack. You can bring the plate of steamed food directly to the table.

Cover the pot. Steam for 10 minutes. Test for doneness. The fish should have lost its translucency and flake easily, but it should be very moist.

Note: You can use this same technique to steam shrimp, crab, clams, mussels, or other seafood. We've included a number of recipes for steamed fish to get you started. Once you try this technique and get the hang of it, you'll agree that it's one of the easiest ways to prepare delicious fish.

Makes 1 serving

Oriental Ginger Fish

This recipe is meant to serve four. But you can use just ¼ pound of fish, make the whole recipe of sauce, and have the sauce ready to go for the next time you're in the mood for this tasty treat.

2 tablespoons peanut oil
2 teaspoons grated fresh ginger
2 teaspoons dry sherry
1 tablespoon black bean sauce (optional)
¼ teaspoon hot pepper sauce (optional)
1 pound fresh cod, whitefish, or rockfish fillets
2 green onions, sliced into 3-inch slivers

Follow the general directions for steaming beginning on page 194. Mix the ingredients except the fish and onion in a small bowl. Place the fish on a plate that can be used in the steamer, spread the sauce mixture over the fish, and top with slivers of green onions. Steam for 10 minutes.

Makes 4 servings

Steamed Spinach and Salmon

If there was ever a dish that proved a diet can be delicious, this is the one. It's beautiful to serve and wonderful to eat. What a way to lose and maintain weight! The recipe serves four persons, but you can reduce the ingredients to serve yourself.

½ cup chopped onion
2 tablespoons olive oil
½ teaspoon each fennel seeds, rosemary leaves, salt, pepper
1 bunch fresh spinach, cleaned and stemmed (see page 184)
1 pound fresh salmon steak
Lemon wedges

Follow the general directions for steaming on page 194–195. Combine the onion, oil, and seasonings in a small bowl. Place the spinach leaves on the steamer rack, put the salmon on top of the spinach, and cover with the seasonings mixture. Steam for 10 minutes. Serve with lemon wedges.

Makes 4 servings

Citrus Seasoned Steamed Fish

The aromas generated by this dish will have mouths watering throughout the house. You can vary the flavor by using different types of citrus: orange, lime, or lemon peel. Or you can combine the three. You'll find that this will become one of your favorite ways to remain faithful to the diet.

¼ cup fresh herbs, minced: basil, dill, or as available
2 teaspoons fresh grated citrus peel (orange, lemon, or lime)
1 tablespoon olive oil
1 pound fresh cod, whitefish, sea bass, or rockfish fillets

Follow the general directions for steaming on page 194–195. Combine the herbs with the grated peel and olive oil. Spread the mixture evenly over both sides of the fish. Steam for 10 minutes

Makes 4 servings

Shrimps 'n' Scallops on the Barbie

You can use this recipe with any fish or seafood combination you wish. It doesn't call for vegetables, but if you want to skewer some veggies, just double the marinade ingredients. Skewer the veggies separately, since they take longer to cook than shrimp or scallops.

Skewering Ingredients:
1 pound assorted seafood: shrimp, large sea scallops, fish

Marinade:
½ cup chicken broth
1 tablespoon each: lime, lemon, orange juice, cider vinegar
2 tablespoons canola oil
¼ teaspoon oregano
3 tablespoons finely chopped parsley
3 cloves garlic, minced
½ teaspoon each: salt and white pepper

Peel and devein shrimp. Rinse scallops. Cut fish into chunks. Mix the marinade ingredients in a large plastic food storage bag. Marinate the seafood in the refrigerator for 2 to 3 hours. Skewer the seafood alternately, and broil or grill until shrimp and scallops lose their translucency. Do not overcook these delicate foods.

Makes 4 servings

Fish in Foil

This recipe goes well with aluminum-wrapped sweet potatoes and asparagus.

4 whole trout, baby salmon, *or* other small fish
1 onion, sliced into thin rings
¼ cup finely chopped parsley
1 lemon
Salt and pepper

Rinse fish and place each on a 12-inch-long sheet of aluminum foil. Divide the onion and parsley among the fish, placing in cavity and over the outside. Squeeze lemon into cavity and over fish. Salt and pepper to taste. Wrap and seal fish in the foil. Roast for 15 minutes.

Makes 4 servings

Poached Salmon with Green Sauce

Court Bouillon:
1 quart water
Juice of ½ lemon
2 small carrots, sliced thin
1 small onion, sliced thin
2 bay leaves
6 peppercorns
1 teaspoon salt (optional)

Salmon:
2 salmon fillets, about 7 ounces each

Green Sauce:
¼ cup nonfat sour cream
1½ tablespoons nonfat mayonnaise
¼ teaspoon salt (optional)
½ teaspoon white vinegar
1 green onion, chopped fine
5 tablespoons chopped fresh dill or 2 tablespoons dried
Parsley and lemon for garnish

Place all court bouillon ingredients in a shallow flameproof casserole and heat on stovetop to boiling. Simmer for 10 minutes. Slice remaining lemon half into thin circular slices. Place salmon in casserole, spoon ingredients over the fillets, and top with sliced lemon. Cover with a piece of waxed paper and bake in a preheated 350°F oven for 20 minutes. Prepare the sauce in advance or while salmon poaches. Simply place all ingredients in a blender and whirl.

Makes 1 to 2 servings

Cajun Blackening Seasoning

If you like the bite of Cajun cooking, there's no better place to do blackened fish or chicken breasts than over the coals outdoors. You'll want to get the coals as hot as they'll get and then spread them out flat in the grill or barbecue pit. Put a cast iron skillet right on top of the coals and let it get as hot as Hades. When you slap the fish or chicken down on the skillet, a huge cloud of smoke will form— something you won't want inside your house.

You can buy blackening seasoning in virtually any supermarket or fish store. Chef Paul Prudhomme, who invented the concept of blackening at his New Orleans restaurant K-Paul, has his own Magic brand of seasonings on the market. But you can save money and avoid the high salt content by putting together your own blackening seasonings.

    1 tablespoon paprika
    1 teaspoon each: garlic powder, onion powder, cayenne pepper
    ¾ teaspoon black pepper
    ½ teaspoon each: ground thyme, oregano, dried basil
    2 teaspoons salt (optional)
    1½ pounds of fish or 4 boneless chicken breasts
    Margarine

Sprinkle seasonings liberally over the fish fillets or chicken breasts. Put a pat of margarine on each fillet, and slap onto the smoking-hot cast iron skillet. Sear for 2 minutes, then turn, using another pat of margarine to blacken the other side for 2 minutes. (You can substitute Pam for margarine to save extra fat grams, but it doesn't work quite as well.)

You can skewer practically any kind of food to cook over the coals, or under the broiler. Different marinades provide flavor variety, and everything can be prepared well ahead of time. This is also a terrific way to enjoy extra servings of vegetables.

Makes 4 servings

POULTRY DISHES

Along with fish, poultry dishes should be among your principal choices of entrees. A 3½-ounce serving of roast chicken breast without the skin provides only 173 calories, 4.5 grams of fat, and no carbohydrate. A similar piece of turkey breast supplies 157 calories and a mere 3.2 grams of fat. Both supply generous amounts of protein. The calorie and fat contents soar, however, when you don't remove the skin. Chicken climbs to 222 calories and 10.9 grams of fat. Turkey goes up to 197 calories and 8.3 grams of fat.

Other types of poultry, while still devoid of carbohydrate as is all meat, have higher amounts of fat and calories. Roast duck with the skin has 337 calories and 28.4 grams of fat in a 3½-ounce serving. Goose contains 238 calories and 21.9 grams of fat in the same size serving.

Now we'll be the first to admit that having a piece of plain, roast chicken or turkey two or three times a week can become boring. We've all heard the jokes about the Thanksgiving turkey that stays around for weeks, far outliving its welcome on the dinner table. So you'll want to try as many ways as possible to prepare white-meat poultry. These recipes will please your taste buds. Look for other recipes in magazines. The ground beef in most recipes can be replaced by ground poultry. Just be certain the carbohydrate count stays low so you can remain in ketosis.

Recipes that call for ground poultry meat are based on ground white meat of chicken or turkey. If your store does not carry the ground meat, ask your butcher to skin and bone a few breasts and grind them. Check packaged ground meat to be sure it is white meat and contains no unwanted and unexpected fat and carbohydrate.

Italian Poultry Burger

1 pound ground chicken *or* turkey breast
4 tablespoons unprocessed bran
1 teaspoon finely minced parsley
¼ teaspoon oregano
¼ teaspoon marjoram
1 garlic clove, finely minced
3 tablespoons chopped onions

Combine all the ingredients and form into four burgers. Grill or broil for about 3 minutes on each side.

Makes 4 servings

Poultry Meatloaf

Here's a recipe the whole family will love. You can make it as one large loaf or four individual loaves. You may also wish to make an extra loaf to keep in the freezer for another time.

1 pound ground chicken *or* turkey breast
1 beaten egg *or* egg substitute
4 tablespoons unprocessed bran
1 tablespoon Worcestershire sauce
½ teaspoon Dijon mustard
1 large garlic clove, finely minced
3 tablespoons finely minced onion
¼ teaspoon each sage, black pepper, marjoram, celery salt
1 teaspoon salt

Combine all the ingredients and form into one large loaf or four small loaves. Bake in a preheated 350°F oven for 1¼ hours. Use a meat thermometer to check for doneness (175°F).

Makes 4 servings

Chinese Stir-Fry

Have you ever wondered how a Chinese restaurant can offer so many different dishes? It's simply a matter of making different combinations of many ingredients, and you can do the same in your kitchen. You won't become bored with your diet program if you emphasize Chinese stir-fry cooking. You can have a different dish every day.

One day cook up some scallops with broccoli, another day have chicken with broccoli, and yet on another day make chicken with bamboo shoots and bell pepper. The possibilities are endless, and they can be varied even more by changing seasonings. Oyster sauce and five-spice powder provide unusual tastes. You can change the flavor of a dish entirely by omitting those seasonings and adding two cloves of garlic. A teaspoon of Chinese hot chili sauce will turn any combination of food into a fiery concoction. Chinese black bean sauce is particularly good with seafood.

Chinese cooking is both low in calories and healthful. You'll want to enjoy such dishes frequently, both when losing weight and when maintaining that loss. If you don't already have one, treat yourself to a good wok. Who deserves it more?

Italian Meatballs

1 pound ground chicken *or* turkey breast
2 tablespoons finely minced green pepper
2 tablespoons finely minced onion
1 tablespoon grated Parmesan cheese
1 large garlic clove, finely minced
4 tablespoons unprocessed bran
¼ teaspoon each oregano, black pepper, thyme, salt
Vegetable oil spray

Combine all the ingredients except cooking spray and form into 12 meatballs. Fry in nonstick pan sprayed with vegetable oil spray.

Makes 4 servings

Oriental Poultry Burgers

Here's a delicious twist on the standard burgers you've been eating. Try serving these Oriental burgers with bean sprouts or Chinese pea pods.

1 pound ground chicken *or* turkey breast
4 tablespoons unprocessed bran
1 tablespoon soy sauce
½ teaspoon freshly grated ginger
½ teaspoon powdered coriander

Combine all the ingredients and form into four burgers. Grill or broil the burgers for about 3 minutes on each side.

Makes 4 servings

Florentine Chicken

1 tablespoon chicken bouillon
¼ teaspoon each thyme, salt, pepper
1 cup fresh spinach *or* ½ cup thawed frozen spinach
4 ounces chicken breast (skinless and boneless)
1 tablespoon grated Parmesan cheese

Combine the bouillon with the seasonings and mix with the spinach. Place the seasoned spinach on the bottom of a casserole and place the chicken breast on top of the bed of spinach. Sprinkle with cheese. Cover. Bake in a preheated 350°F oven for 30 minutes.

Makes 1 serving

Poultry Burgers

Why not prepare several burgers and store them in the freezer? That way you can pop one out whenever you don't have the time for elaborate dinner preparations. When cooking, make an extra patty you can have later in the week as a sandwich for lunch.

4 ounces ground chicken *or* turkey breast
1 tablespoon finely minced onion
1 tablespoon unprocessed bran
¼ teaspoon paprika
¼ teaspoon salt
Lettuce leaves
Dijon mustard
Thinly sliced onion rings

Combine the poultry, minced onion, bran, paprika, and salt and form into a burger. Grill or broil the burger but be sure not to overcook. Count on half the time needed for beef, about 3 minutes on each side. Serve on large leaves of lettuce with a dab of Dijon mustard and some raw onion rings.

Makes 1 serving

Turkey Cutlets

Practically any veal recipe can be duplicated deliciously with turkey, at a real saving in fat and calories. Have your butcher skin and bone a large turkey breast and cut it into cutlets weighing 4 ounces each. You can package them separately and have them ready in the freezer for whenever you'd like to cook them. You may want to prepare two cutlets so you can enjoy one of them for lunch that week. Serve the cutlet as a sandwich on two large lettuce leaves with a dab of Dijon mustard.

    4 ounces turkey cutlet
    1 beaten egg *or* egg substitute
    2 tablespoons unprocessed bran
    Vegetable oil spray

Dip turkey cutlet first into the egg or egg substitute and then into the bran to coat. Allow the coated cutlet to set for about 10 minutes; this helps to keep the coating firmer and less likely to crumble off when cooking. Spray pan with vegetable oil spray. Sauté the cutlet until crisp, about 3 minutes per side.

Makes 1 serving

Chicken Cacciatore

    4 ounces chicken breast (boneless and skinless)
    ¼ cup chicken bouillon
    1 tablespoon each chopped onion, green pepper, tomato,
      mushrooms
    1 garlic clove, finely minced
    1 bay leaf
    ¼ teaspoon each oregano, thyme, salt

Cut chicken into strips. Sauté in a nonstick pan with the chicken bouillon until the chicken is no longer pink. Add vegetables and seasonings. Simmer until tender.

Note: If you increase the amount of vegetables to a total of 1 cup raw, this dish will then provide both your protein and vegetable allowances for a meal.

Makes 1 serving

Chinese Chicken Stir-Fry

4 ounces chicken breast (skinless and boneless)
2 tablespoons chicken bouillon
1 tablespoon oyster sauce
1 teaspoon soy sauce
1 tablespoon unprocessed bran
¼ teaspoon Chinese five-spice powder
1 cup total raw vegetables: bean sprouts, water chestnuts,
    mushrooms, pea pods, broccoli, bamboo shoots

Cut chicken into small strips. Chop vegetables into bite-size pieces. Combine 1 tablespoon of the bouillon with the remaining ingredients to make a sauce. Heat the remaining tablespoon of bouillon to boiling in a large skillet or wok. Stir-fry the chicken until it loses its pink color. Remove it from the skillet. Stir-fry the vegetables until tender. Return the chicken to the skillet along with combined sauce. Heat to boiling, stirring. Serve.

Note: This dish includes both the protein food and the vegetable for a meal.

Makes 1 serving

Chicken Breast Mexicali

This dish is a great example of how a recipe can be adapted to suit your tastes and to provide variety as well. While the recipe calls for chicken breast, you can use the same ingredients and technique with fish fillets, turkey, or other kinds of meats. You'll be surprised at how easy it is to whip up such a festive dish even when time is short.

Vegetable oil spray
4 ounces chicken breast (skinless and boneless)
1 garlic clove, finely minced
1 tablespoon chopped green pepper
1 tablespoon chopped onion
1 tablespoon chopped tomato
Hot pepper sauce to taste
1 tablespoon chopped cilantro
1 tablespoon chicken bouillon

Coat a nonstick pan with vegetable oil spray and heat. Sauté the chicken breast along with minced garlic clove until garlic begins to turn golden. Mix the remaining ingredients and pour over the chicken. Cover. Simmer gently for 20 minutes.

Makes 1 serving

Chicken Curry

This dish is especially delicious if you add a part of your daily allotment of fruit to it. Try it with 2 tablespoons of chopped apple, pineapple, or pear. You might also add your meal's selection of vegetables when you cover and simmer the chicken. Just add an extra tablespoon of chicken bouillon.

4 ounces chicken breast (skinless and boneless)
2 tablespoons chicken bouillon
2 tablespoons chopped onion
1 large garlic clove, finely minced
¼ teaspoon curry powder (more if you like spicy food)
¼ teaspoon paprika

Cut the chicken into thin strips. Sauté in a nonstick pan with the chicken bouillon until white. Combine the remaining ingredients and pour over chicken. Cover. Simmer for 20 minutes or until fork tender.

Makes 1 serving

Green Chili Chicken Stew*

Miss the taste of Mexican food? Try this for your green chili fix!

8 ounces boneless, skinless chicken breast, cubed
½ cup chopped onion
1 to 2 whole green Anaheim chilies, peeled and chopped
1 cup chicken bouillon
Chopped, fresh cilantro, to taste
Cumin to taste
Salt and pepper to taste
1 tablespoon flour to thicken slightly (optional)

Brown chicken in skillet. Add onions and sauté lightly. Add green chili, bouillon, cilantro, and spices. Stir well. Add enough flour to thicken to your taste. Simmer 5 to 10 minutes. Serve in a bowl.

Makes 2 servings

Yummy Chicken and Mushrooms*

8 ounces boneless, skinless chicken breast, cut into strips
½ cup chopped onion
1 cup chicken bouillon
1 tablespoon flour to thicken slightly (optional)
1 cup quartered mushrooms
Salt and pepper to taste
Toss in your favorite spices for different flavors.

Brown chicken in skillet, add onions, and sauté lightly. Add bouillon and optional flour. Simmer gently for 5 to 10 minutes. Add mushrooms just to heat. Season. Serve immediately.

We thank our patient Trudy Warm for contributing these recipes she developed. Also, a special thanks to Elliott Koretz, Joanie Yeoman, Shirley Miller, Julie Hawkins, Joanne Montenaro, and Linda Cohen for the new recipes.

Makes 2 servings

Chicken à l'Orange

4 ounces diet orange soda
⅛ teaspoon each basil, rosemary, sage, salt, thyme
4 ounces chicken breast (skinless and boneless)
1 tablespoon each coarsely chopped onion and mushrooms

Mix the soda with the seasonings. Place the chicken in a small casserole dish and pour the soda mixture over it. Sprinkle onions and mushrooms over the chicken. Cover. Bake in a preheated 350°F oven for 30 minutes.

Makes 1 serving

Sautéed Chicken Breast

You'll never believe this dish is low in calories. The buttery flavor is a real treat.

4 ounces chicken breast (skinless and boneless)
2 tablespoons chicken bouillon
1 teaspoon lemon juice
¼ teaspoon imitation butter extract
¼ teaspoon dry mustard
⅛ teaspoon each powdered ginger and nutmeg

Cut the chicken into small strips. Sauté in 1 tablespoon of chicken bouillon until white. Combine the remaining bouillon with the other ingredients and pour over the chicken. Cover. Simmer for 20 minutes.

Makes 1 serving

Homemade Turkey Broth

Turkey carcass and scraps
3 quarts cold water (or water to cover)
1 teaspoon salt

Place turkey carcass and scraps in the water. Add the salt. Bring to a simmer and skim off any fat that rises to the surface. Simmer at least

3 hours. Do not allow to come to a fast boil, and skim several times. Allow to cool and skim again.

Makes 3 servings

Chicken Cobb Salad

The original Cobb salad was served at the Brown Derby restaurant in Hollywood many years ago. This version calls for ingredients to be coarsely chopped and mixed with dressing.

8 large lettuce leaves
6 cups head lettuce, chopped
1 small tomato, chopped
2 green onions, chopped
1 cup red cabbage, chopped
2 cups cooked chicken breast, chopped
4 hard-cooked eggs, chopped
½ cup Low-Cal Vinaigrette dressing (see page 216)

Arrange the lettuce leaves on the plates. Mix all the remaining ingredients and mound on the lettuce leaves.

Note: This dish includes both the protein food and the vegetable for a meal.

Makes 4 servings

Turkey or Chicken Salad

6 cups fresh spinach leaves
Grapefruit and orange segments
½ cup finely chopped bell pepper
2 cups cooked chicken *or* turkey breast, cubed
½ teaspoon dry mustard
½ teaspoon paprika
1 garlic clove, finely minced
½ teaspoon poppy seeds
¼ cup low fat mayonnaise

On each plate, arrange spinach leaves to form a bed. Decorate the edges of the plate with alternating grapefruit and orange segments. Mix the remaining ingredients and place a scoop of the mixture in the center of each plate.

Note: This dish includes both the protein food and fruit for a meal.

Makes 2 servings

Lemon-Mustard Chicken Wings

Though this recipe works best with wings, you can use other chicken parts. Also consider using turkey wings. This recipe serves four persons, so you can use it for the entire family or cut it down as necessary. You could make half the recipe so you could eat one portion now and save the other for tomorrow.

1 tablespoon Dijon mustard
¼ cup lemon juice
¼ teaspoon lemon pepper
4 garlic cloves, minced
¼ cup corn oil
2 pounds chicken wings

Combine all the ingredients except the chicken to make a basting mixture. Grill or broil the chicken, basting until done, about 20 minutes. Test for doneness by tugging at the wing joint; when the bones separate easily, the chicken is done.

Makes 4 servings

Turkey Chili

The original chili was made without any beans at all. Translated literally, chili con carne means "chili peppers with meat." So let's go back to the basics for this bean- and carbohydrate-free chili.

1 pound ground turkey
1 cup chicken bouillon
½ cup green and red bell peppers, chopped
3 tablespoons chopped onion

2 garlic cloves, finely minced
1 teaspoon salt
1 tablespoon chili powder

In a nonstick pan, cook the turkey until crumbly. Add the remaining ingredients. Cover. Simmer for 30 minutes.

Makes 4 servings

RED MEAT

We've all heard so much about fat and cholesterol in terms of heart disease that many people have cut back considerably on red meat or stopped eating it altogether. While it's true that red meat does contribute substantially to the total fat and cholesterol in the diet, it isn't necessary to eliminate it from the diet completely. Rather it's a matter of learning to use meats in the diet properly. In the past a serving of meat was often a huge slab of well-marbled steak or prime rib. That's just too much of the wrong kind of meat. A more proper serving is about 4 ounces of lean meat. Some cuts of beef are naturally leaner than others. Instead of prime rib, opt for the London broil.

How about pork? Again, see the Appendix for details, but remember that certain cuts, including the tenderloin, loin, and ham, are very low in fat. And look for Smithfield brand pork with even less fat than generic cuts in the supermarket. If your store doesn't stock it, ask the manager to do so for you.

The best advice is to eat a wide variety of foods and enjoy them in moderation. With that in mind, here are some red meat recipes that are light and flavorful.

Beef en Brochette

Keep the fat content low. Your best bet is top sirloin cut in 1½-inch cubes with the fat trimmed off. The oil in all marinades doesn't migrate into the meat very much.

Marinade:
½ cup red wine
¼ cup canola oil

1 teaspoon each Worcestershire sauce and Splenda
1 tablespoon white vinegar
2 tablespoons ketchup
1 clove garlic, minced
½ teaspoon each marjoram and rosemary

Skewering Ingredients:
1 pound top sirloin or other lean beef cut into 1½-inch cubes
16 large fresh mushrooms
2 green bell peppers
2 onions cut in quarters
2 tomatoes cut in quarters

Mix the marinade ingredients together in a large plastic food storage bag. Prepare the meat and vegetables and marinate for 2 to 3 hours in the refrigerator. Skewer the meat and vegetables alternately, and cook over coals or under broiler to preferred doneness.

Makes 4 servings

Javanese Pork Satay

1 pound pork tenderloin in 6 × ¼-inch strips
2 tablespoons peanut butter
½ cup minced onion
1 clove garlic, minced
2 tablespoons lemon juice
1 tablespoon soy sauce
1 tablespoon Splenda
Dash hot pepper sauce

Marinate the tenderloin strips in the mixture formed by blending all the other ingredients for 10 minutes or so. While marinating, soak wooden skewers in water. (This serves two purposes. First, the skewers won't burn if water-logged. Second, the soaked skewers swell in size; as cooking proceeds, they shrink, making it easier to take the meat off.) Thread the pork strips onto the skewers, grill for about 10 minutes, and serve.

Note: The same recipe works quite well with chicken or beef strips.

Makes 4 servings

Herbed Pork and Vegetable Skewers

Marinade:
1 cup beef broth
1 tablespoon lime juice
2 tablespoons canola oil
1 teaspoon each oregano, thyme, onion powder, sage
4 cloves garlic, minced

Skewering Ingredients:
1 pound pork tenderloin, trimmed and cut into cubes
1 pound large mushrooms, ends trimmed
2 bell peppers, cut in eighths (green or mix colors)
2 onions, cut into quarters

Mix the marinade ingredients together in a large plastic food storage bag. Prepare the meat and vegetables and marinate for 2 to 3 hours in the refrigerator. Skewer the meat and vegetables alternately and cook over coals until vegetables are tender and pork is barely pink. Be sure not to overcook the pork.

Makes 4 servings

Beef Orientale

Even if you're in a hurry and cooking just for one, you can make your meal a pleasant one. Here's an approach that works well.

4 ounces filet mignon
4 fresh mushrooms
½ green pepper
¼ onion
1 tablespoon soy sauce
1 teaspoon lemon juice

Cut the meat and vegetables into cubes. Mix the soy sauce and lemon juice, and add the meat and vegetables. Allow to marinate for about 30 minutes. (That's just right to take a shower and get ready for the evening.) To cook, you have a choice—skewer the meat and vegetables and broil (or grill) or quick-fry the meal in a nonstick pan.

Makes 1 serving

Veal and Blue Cheese

Here's just the ticket for jaded taste buds. This is a once-in-a-while treat because of the high fat content of cheese. But as part of a total, varied diet you can enjoy it without guilt. The best part is how easy it is to prepare.

> Vegetable oil spray
> 3 ounces lean veal cutlet
> 1 ounce blue cheese

Coat a nonstick pan with vegetable oil spray and heat. Pound veal thin. Over medium-high heat quickly cook the veal, 3 minutes on one side and 1 minute on the other. Crumble the blue cheese and sprinkle it over the meat. Cover. Cook for 1 minute.

Makes 1 serving

Veal with Lime and Cilantro

> ¼ cup chicken broth
> 1 tablespoon minced cilantro
> ¼ teaspoon salt
> 4 ounces lean veal cutlet
> Juice of ½ lime

In a nonstick pan, bring the broth, cilantro, and salt to a gentle boil. Pound veal cutlets thin and add to pan. Sauté the veal 2 to 3 minutes on each side. Add lime juice. Cover. Simmer for 5 more minutes.

Makes 1 serving

Old-Fashioned Lamb Stew

This recipe can also be made with either beef or pork. But if you haven't had lamb for a while, it's a nice change of pace with a flavor all its own.

> 1 pound lean lamb
> Vegetable oil spray
> 1 cup beef bouillon

1 cup each coarsely chopped celery, rutabaga or parsnips, onion
3 bay leaves
6 juniper berries
2 garlic cloves, minced
1 teaspoon salt
1 teaspoon ground pepper
1 teaspoon marjoram

Cut the lamb into ½- × 1-inch strips. Coat the bottom of a large, heavy pot with vegetable oil spray. Sauté the lamb until browned. Add ½ cup of the beef bouillon. Bring to a boil. Reduce heat, and simmer 30 minutes. Add the remaining bouillon along with vegetables, bay leaves, juniper berries, garlic, salt, pepper, and marjoram. Cover. Cook for 30 minutes or until vegetables are fork tender.

Note: This dish includes both the protein food and the vegetable for a meal.

Makes 4 servings

SALAD DRESSINGS

Even the freshest, crispest salad tastes better with a delicious dressing. But dressings can come packed with fat, calories, and even carbohydrates, ruining your otherwise good intentions. This is another example of how important it is to read the labels of food products. One oil and vinegar dressing may contain 0.6 grams of carbohydrate per tablespoon. But in another, the carbohydrate content may rise to 6.6 grams. That can be just enough to get you out of ketosis and into trouble.

You'll want to watch the calorie and fat content as well as the level of carbohydrate in bottled dressings and packaged mixes. Ranch dressing prepared with regular mayonnaise has only 0.6 grams of carbohydrate per tablespoon but 100 calories and 11 grams of fat.

There are some excellent dressings on the market that are low in calories, carbohydrates, and fat. Look for El Molino Herbal Secrets, Mrs. Pickford's Herb Magic, Pritikin, and Skinny Haven dressings in your supermarket and health-food store. Skinny Haven is particularly convenient because the dressings come in individual packets.

You can easily carry one with you when you go out to dinner and enjoy your salad without guilt.

Homemade salad dressings are best of all. They're easy to prepare and store well, so you can keep two or three kinds in your refrigerator.

Low-Cal Vinaigrette

½ cup water
2 tablespoons oil
2 tablespoons fresh lemon juice
4 tablespoons cider vinegar
2 garlic cloves, minced
1 teaspoon Dijon mustard
1 teaspoon minced fresh basil
1 teaspoon minced fresh chives
1 teaspoon salt
1 teaspoon pepper (freshly ground if possible)

Blend all the ingredients together and store in the refrigerator.

Vinaigrette Variations:
Exclude the garlic and herbs and add other ingredients as
    follows.

Dill Vinaigrette: 1 tablespoon minced fresh dill
Parsley Vinaigrette: 2 tablespoons minced fresh parsley
Curry Vinaigrette: 1 teaspoon curry powder, 1 teaspoon
    ground coriander
Mexican Vinaigrette: 2 tablespoons fresh cilantro

Makes 1 cup (each serving is 1 tablespoon)

DESSERTS

These are delicious and low in carbs, which is hard to find.

Ruth's Low Carb Mini Cheesecake

Each cheesecake is 2–3 carbs. Enjoy them and eat sparingly. They go great with a cup of Sugar Free, Decaffeinated Suisse Mocha coffee by General Foods International.

Crust:
4 tablespoons butter
¾ cup almond meal

Filling:
2 egg whites
12 packets Splenda
2 (8-ounce) packages of cream cheese (1 low fat, 1 nonfat), softened
1 teaspoon vanilla
Scant amount of sweetener

Melt butter and add to almond meal. Beat egg whites until soft peaks form. Add sweetener. Beat cheese until soft and creamy. Fold egg whites into cream cheese. Add vanilla. Place 12 foil cups in muffin tin. Divide crust mixture between 12 muffin cups and pat down gently. Spoon in filling. Bake in a preheated 350°F oven for 15–17 minutes or until center is firm. Remove from oven and cool. Refrigerate 2 hours or overnight before serving.

Makes 12

Angel Bites

5 egg whites
⅓ cup Splenda
1½ teaspoons vanilla
Pinch of salt

Beat egg whites until frothy. Add Splenda, vanilla, and salt. Beat mixture until stiff peaks form. Drop by the spoonful onto cookie sheets. Bake in a preheated 350°F oven for 10–15 minutes or until golden brown.

Makes 16–24 bites (6 per serving)

Gelatin Desserts and Snacks

Many patients find sugar-free gelatin (sweetened with NutraSweet) to be an absolute lifesaver in dieting and in maintaining their weight loss whenever they crave a sweet for dessert or a snack. Experiment with different flavors and serve it different ways. Be sure to keep a supply in the refrigerator at all times. Here are just a few suggestions.

Checkerboard Gelatin

Prepare two colors of sugar-free gelatin, lemon and lime, for example, according to the directions on the package. Pour into flat pans and allow to set. Cut into 1-inch cubes. You can mix the cubes together in wine goblets to make a colorful, attractive treat. Or stick toothpicks into the cubes to enjoy as finger foods.

Makes 6 servings

Gelatin Salad

Stir in a variety of shredded greens before allowing the gelatin to set. Make individual salads in small bowls and glasses or a large salad in a serving bowl. You can form shapes using molds for a festive touch at the table. Dream up all kinds of combinations.

Lemon gelatin with radicchio
Orange gelatin with shredded lettuce
Lime gelatin with strips of spinach
Lemon gelatin with shredded celery, radishes

Note: Any combination such as these will use only a small portion of your daily allotment of greens. Remember that you're permitted the equivalent of one head of lettuce daily.

Gelatin on a Stick

Many of the low calorie frozen confections available today have a large amount of carbohydrates in each serving. Sugar-free gelatin pops are a wonderful easy-to-make substitute.

Spray the inside of small tubular glasses with a bit of vegetable oil spray. Champagne flutes and cordial glasses work well. Prepare the gelatin according to package directions. Pour the gelatin into the glasses and allow to set. Insert popsicle sticks when you remove the gelatin from the glasses. The light spray of oil will let the gelatin slide out easily. Kids will love this idea.

Gelatin "Cookies"

If you've ever cut out cookies during the holidays, you know how much fun it can be. Why not bring out your cookie cutters and use them with gelatin?

Make the gelatin in shallow pans, filled to about the height of cutters. You can have green Christmas trees and red Santas even in July.

COMPOSITION OF COMMONLY CONSUMED FOODS AND BEVERAGES

The following lists of foods show their caloric, carbohydrate, fat, and protein content. They should serve as a guide during your weight loss, stabilization, and maintenance programs—in other words, for the rest of your life. You don't have to memorize the exact composition of each food. The important thing is to be aware of the approximate amounts of calories, carbohydrates, and fats in what you eat.

Take a few minutes to glance through the lists now. As you plan your meals, review the food composition from time to time. We think you'll be surprised—even shocked—at how many calories and how much fat many of the foods contain. One glance at the listings for fast foods should be enough to make anyone vow not to eat them again. Whether you're trying to avoid calories, carbohydrates, or fat, most fast-food restaurants serve up disasters.

These lists can cover only a few items. Don't forget to read the labels of the foods you purchase regularly.

Space limitations prohibit us from supplying data on each and every food you may eat or want to eat. We've tried to provide an overview. For a very extensive compilation of the carbohydrate, fat, and protein contents of a vast number of foods, we recommend *Food Values of Portions Commonly Used* by Jean Pennington. It's available in most bookstores.

Food	Serving Size	Calories	Carbohydrates (g)	Fat (g)	Protein (g)
Alcoholic Beverages					
Beer	12 oz.	148	13.2	0.0	0.9
Beer, light	12 oz.	100	6.0	0.0	0.4
Daiquiri	3½ oz.	122	5.2	0.0	0.0
Liqueurs (54 proof)	1 oz.	97	11.5	0.0	0.0
Manhattan	3½ oz.	164	7.9	0.0	0.0
Martini	3½ oz.	140	0.3	0.0	0.0
Gin, Rum, Vodka, Whiskey, Scotch					
80 proof	1 oz.	65	0.0	0.0	0.0
86 proof	1 oz.	70	0.0	0.0	0.0
90 proof	1 oz.	74	0.0	0.0	0.0
94 proof	1 oz.	77	0.0	0.0	0.0
100 proof	1 oz.	83	0.0	0.0	0.0
Wine					
Champagne	4 oz.	84	3.0	0.0	0.0
Red	3½ oz.	76	2.4	0.0	0.0
White	3½ oz.	80	3.4	0.0	0.0
Carbonated Beverages					
Club soda, mineral water, water	12 oz.	0	0.0	0.0	0.0
Coca-Cola	12 oz.	144	37.5	0.0	0.0
Diet soda	12 oz.	0–2	0.0	0.0	0.0
Dr Pepper	12 oz.	159	40.7	0.0	0.0
Ginger ale	12 oz.	113	29.0	0.0	0.0
Root beer	12 oz.	163	42.2	0.0	0.0
Seven-Up	12 oz.	144	36.0	0.0	0.0
Tonic water	12 oz.	126	31.2	0.0	0.0

Food	Serving Size	Calories	Carbohydrates (g)	Fat (g)	Protein (g)
Candy and Snacks					
Almond Joy	1 oz.	151	18.5	7.8	1.7
Almonds	1 oz.	176	5.5	16.2	5.2
Chunky	12 oz.	143	17.9	7.1	1.9
Corn chips	1 oz.	153	16.6	8.8	1.7
Cracker Jack	1 oz.	114	25.5	1.0	0.8
Hershey's chocolate	1 oz.	160	16.5	9.4	2.2
Jelly beans	10 pieces	66	16.7	0.0	0.0
Marshmallows	1 large	25	6.2	0.0	0.2
Nestle's Crunch	1 oz.	160	19.0	8.0	2.0
Peanuts	1 oz.	170	5.4	14.0	8.6
Popcorn (air popped)	1 cup	54	10.7	0.7	1.8
Potato chips	1 oz.	159	14.0	11.2	3.0
Pretzels	1 oz.	111	22.4	1.0	2.6
Tortilla chips	1 oz.	139	18.6	6.6	2.0
Dairy Foods					
American cheese	1 oz.	106	0.5	8.9	6.3
Buttermilk	1 cup	99	11.7	2.2	8.1
Cheddar cheese	1 oz.	114	0.4	9.4	7.1
Cottage cheese (1 percent fat)	1 cup	164	6.2	2.3	28.0
Cream cheese	1 oz.	99	0.8	9.9	2.1
Gouda cheese	1 oz.	101	0.6	7.8	7.1
Half and half	1 Tbsp.	20	0.6	1.7	0.4
Milk, low fat (1 percent)	1 cup	102	11.7	2.6	8.0
Milk, low fat (2 percent)	1 cup	121	11.7	4.7	8.1
Milk, nonfat (skim)	1 cup	86	11.9	0.4	8.4
Milk, whole	1 cup	150	11.0	8.0	8.0
Monterey Jack cheese	1 oz.	106	0.2	8.6	6.9
Mozzarella cheese (part skim)	1 oz.	72	0.8	4.5	6.9
Swiss cheese	1 oz.	107	1.0	7.8	8.1
Yogurt, fruit	1 cup	225	42.3	2.6	9.0
Yogurt, low fat	1 cup	144	16.0	3.5	11.9
Yogurt, nonfat	1 cup	127	17.4	0.4	13.0

Food	Serving Size	Calories	Carbohydrates (g)	Fat (g)	Protein (g)
Dairy Foods (continued)					
Sour cream	1 Tbsp.	26	0.5	2.5	0.4
Whipping cream	1 Tbsp.	52	0.4	5.6	0.3
Desserts					
Angel food cake	2 oz.	126	35.7	0.1	4.8
Apple pie	4 oz.	282	43.0	11.9	2.4
Boston cream pie	2 oz.	332	54.9	10.3	5.5
Cheesecake (plain)	2 oz.	150	37.8	14.3	6.0
Chocolate chip cookies	2 oz.	230	32.0	13.5	2.5
Custard	½ cup	153	14.7	7.3	7.1
Danish pastry	1 oz.	121	17.4	4.9	1.8
Devil's food cake	2 oz.	233	34.2	10.8	2.6
Doughnut	1 oz.	151	21.7	8.4	4.5
Gelatin (w/NutraSweet)	½ cup	8	0.0	0.0	1.6
Gelatin (sugar)	½ cup	81	18.7	0.0	1.6
Ice cream (10 percent fat)	1 cup	269	31.7	14.3	4.8
Ice cream (16 percent fat)	1 cup	349	32.0	23.7	4.1
Lemon meringue pie	4 oz.	250	42.0	10.0	2.0
Oatmeal cookies	2 oz.	260	34.0	12.0	2.0
Eggs					
Egg substitute	¼ cup	30	1.0	0.0	6.0
Egg white	1 large	16	0.0	0.4	3.4
Whole egg	1 large	79	0.6	5.6	6.1
Fast Foods					
Burger King					
Cheeseburger, regular	1 oz.	350	30.0	17.0	18.0
Cheeseburger, Whopper	1 oz.	740	52.0	45.0	32.0
French fries	1 order	210	25.0	11.0	3.0
Kentucky Fried Chicken					
Chicken sandwich	1	436	33.8	22.5	24.8
Fried chicken, drumstick	1	155	5.1	9.0	13.3

Food	Serving Size	Calories	Carbohydrates (g)	Fat (g)	Protein (g)
Fast Foods (continued)					
Fried chicken, extra crispy thigh	1	343	12.6	23.4	20.4
Long John Silver's					
Fish, batter fried	3 pieces	549	32.0	32.0	32.0
Fish sandwich	1	560	49.0	31.0	22.0
McDonald's					
Egg McMuffin	1	327	31.0	14.8	18.5
Big Mac	1	563	40.6	33.0	25.7
Meat					
Beef composite, cooked and trimmed	3 oz.	192	0.0	9.4	25.0
Round steak, cooked and trimmed	3 oz.	158	0.0	6.0	25.0
Sirloin steak, cooked and trimmed	3 oz.	185	0.0	8.3	26.0
Rib steak, cooked and trimmed	3 oz.	200	0.0	10.9	24.0
Pot roast, cooked and trimmed	3 oz.	205	0.0	9.3	28.0
Tenderloin, cooked and trimmed	3 oz.	183	0.0	8.9	24.0
Ground beef (18 percent fat), cooked and drained	3 oz.	192	0.0	14.4	24.0
Lamb composite, cooked and trimmed	3 oz.	176	0.0	8.1	24.0
Loin chop, cooked and trimmed	3 oz.	188	0.0	8.9	25.0
Rib roast, cooked and trimmed	3 oz.	211	0.0	12.9	22.0
Shank, cooked and trimmed	3 oz.	168	0.0	5.5	28.0
Pork composite, cooked and trimmed	3 oz.	198	0.0	11.1	23.0
Loin chop, cooked and trimmed	3 oz.	219	0.0	12.7	24.0

Food	Serving Size	Calories	Carbohydrates (g)	Fat (g)	Protein (g)
Meat (continued)					
Loin roast, cooked and trimmed	3 oz.	208	0.0	11.7	24.0
Spareribs, cooked and trimmed	3 oz.	338	0.0	25.8	25.0
Tenderloin, cooked and trimmed	3 oz.	141	0.0	4.1	24.0
Breakfast					
Bacon, crisp	3 slices	105	0.3	9.3	4.8
Canadian bacon	1, 1-oz. slice	40	0.0	2.0	5.6
Pork sausage	1, 2-oz. link	265	1.4	21.6	15.1
Luncheon					
Beef bologna	1, 1-oz. slice	80	1.0	7.0	3.0
Ham (5 percent fat)	1, 1-oz. slice	37	0.3	1.4	5.5
Hot dog, beef	1, 2-oz. frank	150	2.0	15.0	6.0
Hot dog, chicken	1, 2-oz. frank	120	4.0	9.0	6.0
Salami, beef	1, 1-oz. link	58	0.6	4.6	3.4
Turkey breast	1, 1-oz. link	20	0.0	0.2	5.0
Poultry					
Chicken, dark, roasted, w/o skin	3½ oz.	205	0. 0	9.7	27.4
Chicken, dark, roasted, w/skin	3½ oz.	253	0.0	15.8	26.0
Chicken, white, roasted, w/o skin	3½ oz.	173	0.0	4.5	30.9
Duck, roasted, w/skin,	3½ oz.	337	0.0	28.4	19.0
Turkey, all, roasted, w/skin	3½ oz.	208	0.0	9.7	28.1
Turkey, dark, roasted, w/o skin	3½ oz.	187	0.0	7.2	28.6
Turkey, white, roasted, w/o skin	3½ oz.	157	0.0	3.2	29.9

Food	Serving Size	Calories	Carbohydrates (g)	Fat (g)	Protein (g)
Fish and Seafood					
Bass, broiled	3½ oz.	228	0.0	2.7	18.9
Clams, canned	3½ oz.	98	0.0	2.5	15.8
Cod, broiled	3½ oz.	162	0.0	0.3	17.6
Fillets, batter fried	2, 6-oz. pieces	440	25.0	31.0	17.0
Fish sticks	4, 3½ oz. pieces	176	6.5	8.9	16.6
Halibut, broiled	3½ oz.	100	0.0	1.2	20.9
Lobster, broiled	3½ oz.	91	0.0	1.9	16.9
Oysters, canned	3½ oz.	76	0.0	2.2	8.5
Salmon, broiled	3½ oz.	182	0.0	7.4	27.0
Salmon, silver, canned	3½ oz.	153	0.0	8.2	18.8
Scallops, steamed	3½ oz.	81	0.0	0.2	15.3
Tuna, canned in oil	3½ oz.	190	0.0	10.0	25.0
Tuna, canned in water	3½ oz.	118	0.0	1.7	26.0
Grains, Breads, and Pasta					
Bagel, water	1	163	30.9	1.4	6.0
Blueberry muffin	1	126	19.5	4.3	2.4
Bread, corn	2 oz.	160	26.0	4.0	4.0
Bread, French	1 slice	70	12.6	1.0	2.4
Bread, rye	1 slice	66	12.0	0.9	2.1
Bread, sourdough	1 slice	68	13.4	0.5	2.5
Bread, wheat	1 slice	66	12.5	0.8	2.2
Bread, white	1 slice	66	11.7	0.9	2.0
Bread crumbs	1 cup	345	64.6	4.0	11.1
English muffin	1 muffin	135	26.2	1.1	4.5
Noodles, cooked	¾ cup	107	20.1	1.2	3.9
Pasta, cooked	¾ cup	150	30.0	0.4	5.1
Rice, cooked	⅓ cup	80	15.0	0.0	3.0
Saltines	2 crackers	26	4.4	0.6	0.6
Triscuits	2 crackers	42	6.2	1.5	0.8
Waffles	1 large	245	25.7	12.6	6.9
Wheat Thins	4 crackers	36	5.0	1.4	0.5

Food	Serving Size	Calories	Carbohydrates (g)	Fat (g)	Protein (g)
		Cereals			
Composite bran cereals	⅓ cup	80	15.0	trace	3.0
Composite cooked cereals	½ cup	80	15.0	trace	3.0
Composite uncooked cereals	¾ cup	80	15.0	trace	3.0
Composite puffed cereals	1½ cups	80	15.0	trace	3.0
Cream of Rice, cooked	¾ cup	95	21.1	0.1	1.6
Cream of Wheat, cooked	¾ cup	100	20.8	0.4	2.9
Oatmeal, cooked	¾ cup	108	18.9	1.8	4.5
All-Bran	1 oz.	71	21.1	0.5	4.0
Cheerios	1 oz.	111	19.6	1.8	4.3
Corn Flakes	1 oz.	110	24.4	0.1	2.3
Frosted Flakes	1 oz.	110	26.0	0.1	1.4
Grape-Nuts	1 oz.	101	23.2	0.1	3.3
Raisin Bran	1 oz.	87	21.4	0.5	2.6
Shredded Wheat (1 biscuit)	1 oz.	83	18.8	0.3	1.8
Wheaties	1 oz.	99	22.6	0.5	2.7
		Fruits			
Composite fresh fruit	½ cup	60	15.0	0.0	trace
Composite dried fruit	¼ cup	60	15.0	0.0	trace
Composite fruit juice	½ cup	60	15.0	0.0	trace
Apple, raw	1, 2-inch	60	15.0	0.0	trace
Applesauce (unsweetened)	½ cup	60	15.0	0.0	trace
Apricots, raw	1, 2-inch	60	15.0	0.0	trace
Apricots, canned	½ cup	60	15.0	0.0	trace
Avocado, California	1 medium	306	12.0	30.0	3.6
Banana	1, 9-inch	60	15.0	0.0	trace
Blackberries, raw	¾ cup	60	15.0	0.0	trace
Blueberries, raw	¾ cup	60	15.0	0.0	trace
Cantaloupe	⅓, 5-inch	60	15.0	0.0	trace
Cantaloupe, cubes	1 cup	60	15.0	0.0	trace
Cherries, raw	½ cup, large	60	15.0	0.0	trace
Cherries, canned	½ cup	60	15.0	0.0	trace
Figs, raw	2, 2-inch	60	15.0	0.0	trace
Fruit cocktail, canned	½ cup	60	15.0	0.0	trace
Grapefruit	½ medium	60	15.0	0.0	trace

Food	Serving Size	Calories	Carbohydrates (g)	Fat (g)	Protein (g)
		Fruits (continued)			
Grapefruit, segments	¾ cup	60	15.0	0.0	trace
Grapes	15 small	60	15.0	0.0	trace
Honeydew melon	⅛ medium	60	15.0	0.0	trace
Honeydew, cubes	1 cup	60	15.0	0.0	trace
Kiwi	1 large	60	15.0	0.0	trace
Mandarin orange segments	¾ cup	60	15.0	0.0	trace
Mango	½ small	60	15.0	0.0	trace
Nectarine	1, ½-inch	60	15.0	0.0	trace
Orange	1, 2½-inch	60	15.0	0.0	trace
Papaya	1 cup	60	15.0	0.0	trace
Peach	1, 2¾-inch	60	15.0	0.0	trace
Peaches, canned	½ cup, 2 halves	60	15.0	0.0	trace
Pear	½ cup, 1 small	60	15.0	0.0	trace
Pears, canned	½ cup, 2 halves	60	15.0	0.0	trace
Pineapple, cubes	¾ cup	60	15.0	0.0	trace
Pineapple, canned	⅓ cup	60	15.0	0.0	trace
Plum, raw	2, 2-inch	60	15.0	0.0	trace
Raspberries, raw	1 cup	60	15.0	0.0	trace
Strawberries, raw	1¼ cups	60	15.0	0.0	trace
Tangerine	2, 2½-inch	60	15.0	0.0	trace
Watermelon, cubes	1¼ cup	60	15.0	0.0	trace
Dried apples	4 rings	60	15.0	0.0	trace
Dried apricots	7 halves	60	15.0	0.0	trace
Dried dates	2½ medium	60	15.0	0.0	trace
Dried figs	1½	60	15.0	0.0	trace
Raisins	2 Tbsp.	60	15.0	0.0	trace
Dried prunes	3 medium	60	15.0	0.0	trace
Apple juice/cider	½ cup	60	15.0	0.0	trace
Cranberry juice	⅓ cup	60	15.0	0.0	trace
Grapefruit juice	½ cup	60	15.0	0.0	trace
Grape juice	⅓ cup	60	15.0	0.0	trace
Orange juice	½ cup	60	15.0	0.0	trace
Pineapple juice	½ cup	60	15.0	0.0	trace
Prune juice	⅓ cup	60	15.0	0.0	trace

Food	Serving Size	Calories	Carbohydrates (g)	Fat (g)	Protein (g)
Vegetables					
Composite cooked vegetable	½ cup	25	5.0	0.0	1.0–5.0
Composite vegetable juice	½ cup	25	5.0	0.0	1.0–2.0
Composite raw vegetable	1 cup	25	5.0	0.0	1.0–2.0
Composite Starchy vegetables					
Beans, cooked	⅓ cup	80	15.0	0.0	3.0
Corn	½ cup	80	15.0	0.0	3.0
Corn on the cob	1, 6-inch cob	80	15.0	0.0	3.0
Lentils, cooked	⅓ cup	80	15.0	0.0	3.0
Lima beans	½ cup	80	15.0	0.0	3.0
Peas, canned/frozen	½ cup	80	15.0	0.0	3.0
Plantain	½ cup	80	15.0	0.0	3.0
Potato, baked	1, 3 oz.	80	15.0	0.0	3.0
Potato, mashed	½ cup	80	15.0	0.0	3.0
Squash	¾ cup	80	15.0	0.0	3.0
Sweet potato	⅓ cup	80	15.0	0.0	3.0
Yam	⅓ cup	80	15.0	0.0	3.0
"Free" Vegetables					
Cabbage, shredded	1 cup	24	5.4	0.0	1.3
Celery, raw	1 stalk	8	2.0	0.0	0.4
Chives raw, chopped	1 Tbsp.	3	0.6	0.0	0.2
Lettuce, butter	1 cup	14	2.5	0.0	1.2
Iceberg	1 cup	13	2.9	0.0	0.9
Romaine	1 cup	18	3.5	0.0	1.3
Parsley, chopped	1 Tbsp.	4	0.8	0.0	0.4
Spinach, raw	1 cup	26	4.3	0.0	3.2

Food	Serving Size	Calories	Carbohydrates (g)	Fat (g)	Protein (g)
Fats and Oils					
Butter	1 Tbsp.	108	0.0	12.2	0.0
Margarine	1 Tbsp.	102	0.0	11.4	0.0
Mayonnaise	1 Tbsp.	99	1.0	11.0	0.2
Mayonnaise, low fat	1 Tbsp.	40	1.0	4.0	0.0
Oil (all types)	1 Tbsp.	120	0.0	13.6	0.0
Salad Dressings					
Blue cheese	1 Tbsp.	77	1.1	8.0	0.7
Buttermilk	1 Tbsp.	58	1.2	5.8	0.5
Caesar	1 Tbsp.	70	1.0	7.0	0.0
French	1 Tbsp.	67	2.7	6.4	0.1
Green Goddess	1 Tbsp.	68	1.2	7.0	0.1
Italian	1 Tbsp.	69	1.5	7.1	0.1
Italian, creamy	1 Tbsp.	52	2.7	4.5	0.1
Oil and vinegar	1 Tbsp.	103	6.6	8.5	0.1
Thousand Island	1 Tbsp.	59	2.4	5.6	0.1

BIBLIOGRAPHY

Bjorntorp, P. "Abdominal Obesity and the Development of Noninsuline-Dependent Diabetes Mellitus." *Diabetes Metabolism Reviews* 4 (1988): 615–22.

Bliss, Michael. *The Discovery of Insulin*. Chicago: University of Chicago Press, 1982.

Bohmer, M. et al. "Long Term Metformin Use Is Associated with Decreased Risk of Breast Cancer." *Diabetes Care* 33 (2010): 1304.

DeFronzo, R. A., and E. Ferrannini. "Insulin Resistance: A Multifaceted Syndrome Responsible for NIDDM, Obesity, Hypertension, Dyslipidemia, and Atherosclerotic Cardiovascular Disease." *Diabetes Care* 14 (1991): 173–94.

Ezrin, C. "Childhood Diabetes." *University of Toronto Medical Journal* 26 (1949): 233–39.

Ezrin, C., J. M. Salter, M. A. Ogryzlo, and C. H. Best. "the Clinical and Metabolic Effects of Glucagon." *Canadian Medical Association Journal* 78 (1958): 96–98.

Ezrin, C., J. O. Godden, and R. Volpe. *Systematic Endocrinology, 2d ed.* New York: Harper & Row, 1979.

Ezrin, C., and K. Caron. *Deperately Seeking Serotonin, Your Fat Can Make You Think*. New York: McGraw-Hill, 2001.

Ezrin, C., and P. J. Moloney. "Resistance to Insulin Due to Neutralizing Antibodies." *Journal of Clinical Endocrinology and Metabolism* 19 (1959): 1055–68.

Flegal, K. M., et al. "Prevalence and Trends in Obesity Among U.S. Adults 1999–2008." *Journal of the American Medical Association* 303(3) (2010): 235–41.

Flier, J. S., and J. K. Ermquest. "A Good Night's Sleep: Future Antidote to the Obesity Epidemic." *Annals of Internal Medicine* 141 (2004): 885–86.

Hartmann, E. "Effects of L-Tryptophan on Sleepiness and on Sleep." *Journal of Psychiatric Research* 17(2) (1982–83): 107–13.

Lorenzo, C., et al. "A1C Between 5.7 and 6.4% as a Marker for Identifying Pre-Diabetes, Insulin Sensitivity and Secretion and Cardiovascular Risk Factors." *Diabetes Care* 33 (2010): 2104–9.

Manson, J. E., P. J. Skerrett, P. Greenland, and T. B. Vanltallie. "The Escalating Pandemics of Obesity and Sedentary Lifestyle: A Call to Action for Clincians." *Archives of Internal Medicine* 164(3) (2004): 249–58.

Moller, D. E., and J. S. Flier. "Insulin Resistance: Mechanisms, Syndromes, and Implications." *New England Journal of Medicine* 325 (1991): 938–48.

Muldoon, M., R. H. Mackey, N. Korytkowski, et al. "The Metabolic Syndrome Is Associated with Reduced Central Serontoninergic Responsivity in Healthy Community Volunteers." *Journal of Clincial Endocrinology and Metabolism* 91 (2006): 718–21.

Pacy, P. J., J. Webster, and J. S. Garrow. "Exercise and Obesity." *Sports Medicine* 3 (1986): 89–113.

Reaven, G. N. "Role of Insulin Resistance in Human Disease." *Diabetes* 37 (1988): 1595–1607.

Ronnemaa, T., M. Laakso, K. Pyörälä, V. Kallio, and P. Puukka. "High Fasting Plasma Insulin as an Indicator of Coronary Heart Disease in Non-Insulin Diabetic Patients and Non-Diabetic Subjects." *Arteriosclerosis and Thrombosis* 11 (1991): 80–90.

Salter, J. M., C. Ezrin, J. C. Laidlaw, and A. G. Gornall. "Metabolic Effects of Glucagon in Human Subjects." *Metabolism* 9 (1959): 753–68.

Singh, M., C. L. Drake, T. Roehrs, et al. "The Association Between Obesity and Short Sleep Duration: A Population-Based Study." *Journal of Clinical Sleep Medicine* 1(4) (2005): 247–63.

Spiegel, K., E. Tesali, P. Plenev, and E. Van Cauter. "Brief Communication: Sleep Curtailment in Healthy Young Man Is Associated with Decreased Leptin Levels, Elevated Ghrelin Levels and Increased Hunger and Appetite." *Annals in Internal Medicine* 141 (2004): 846–50.

Spiegel, K., E. Van Cauter, and R. Leproult. "Impact of Sleep Debt on Metabolic and Endocrine Function." *Lancet* 354(9188) (1999): 1435–39.

Wadden, T. A., and A. J. Stunkard. "Social and Psychological Consequences of Obesity." *Annals in Internal Medicine* 103(6) (1985): 1062–67.

Walsh, J. K., and P. J. Schweitzer. "Ten-Year Trends in Pharmocological Treatment of Insomnia." *Sleep* 22 (1999): 3, 371–75.

Ware, J. C., and J. D. Pittard. "Increased Deep Sleep After Trazodone Use: A Double-Blind Placebo-Controlled Study in Healthy Young Adults." *Journal of Clincial Psychiatry* 51(9) (1990; suppl.): 18–22.

Wurtman, R. J. "Nutrients That Modify Brain Function." *Scientific American* 246 (1982): 50–59.

Wurtman, R. J., and J. J. Wurtman. "Brain Serotonin Carbohydrate Craving, Obesity and Depression." *Obesity Research* 3 (1995): 5, 477–80.

INDEX